J. Wickham (John Wickham) Legg, Henry Jones

A Guide to the Examination of the Urine

J. Wickham (John Wickham) Legg, Henry Jones

A Guide to the Examination of the Urine

ISBN/EAN: 9783742831378

Manufactured in Europe, USA, Canada, Australia, Japa

Cover: Foto ©Lupo / pixelio.de

Manufactured and distributed by brebook publishing software
(www.brebook.com)

J. Wickham (John Wickham) Legg, Henry Jones

A Guide to the Examination of the Urine

A GUIDE

TO THE

EXAMINATION OF THE URINE

BY

J. WICKHAM LEGG

FELLOW OF THE ROYAL COLLEGE OF PHYSICIANS OF LONDON; FORMERLY
ASSISTANT PHYSICIAN TO ST. BARTHOLOMEW'S HOSPITAL AND LEC-
TURER ON PATHOLOGICAL ANATOMY IN THE MEDICAL SCHOOL

SEVENTH EDITION

EDITED AND REVISED BY

H. LEWIS JONES, M.A., M.D.

MEMBER OF THE ROYAL COLLEGE OF PHYSICIANS; MEDICAL OFFICER
IN CHARGE OF THE ELECTRICAL DEPARTMENT IN
ST. BARTHOLOMEW'S HOSPITAL

PHILADELPHIA
P. BLAKISTON, SON & Co.
No. 1012 WALNUT STREET
1893

PREFACE TO THE SEVENTH EDITION.

THE present edition has been carefully revised throughout; the arrangement of the sections has been slightly modified, and some parts have been rewritten. About twenty pages of fresh matter, and twelve new illustrations have been added; the latter include several reproductions by photography of actual specimens of urinary crystals.

H. LEWIS JONES, M.D.

9 Upper Wimpole St., W.
Sept. 5th, 1893.

CONTENTS.

INTRODUCTION.

THIS little work is intended to supply the clinical clerk and student of medicine with a concise guide to the recognition of the more important characters of the urine; and from its small size to serve as a companion at the bedside to the busy practitioner, who may be unable to consult the larger works on the subject. A plan for the examination of the urine, step by step, has been given, with an account of the method for ascertaining the nature of those alterations that are most frequently seen in disease. An appendix has been added in which the manner of estimating the urea, chlorides, phosphates, sugar, &c., by volumetric or other rapid analysis has been described.

A GUIDE

TO THE

EXAMINATION OF THE URINE.

TABLE OF THE COMPOSITION OF THE URINE.

THE following table gives the average daily quantity of the chief urinary constituents.*

Water	1500 c.c.	52½ ounces
Solids	72·03 grms.	1110·79 grs.
Urea	33·18 ,,	512·4 ,,
Kreatinin	0·91 ,,	14·0 ,,
Uric Acid	0·55 ,,	8·57 ,,
Hippuric acid	0·40 ,,	6·16 ,,
" Pigment and Extractive "	10·00 ,,	154·0 ,,
Sulphuric Acid	2·01 ,,	30·98 ,,
Phosphoric Acid	3·16 ,,	48·8 ,,
Chlorine	7·00 ,,	107·8 ,,
Ammonia	0·77 ,,	11·8 ,,
Potassium	2·50 ,,	38·5 ,,
Sodium	11·09 ,,	170·78 ,,
Calcium	0·26 ,,	4·0 ,,
Magnesium	0·20 ,,	3·0 ,,

* Adapted from Kirkes' *Physiology*. Thirteenth Edition.

In order that the examination of the urine may be made on a definite plan, the following scheme is recommended to the student.

The order of examination that is here given should be followed always; the details of each operation are described on the page referred to at the end of each paragraph. Notes should be taken of each observation.

PRELIMINARY SCHEME FOR THE EXAMINATION OF THE URINE.

I. Observe the colour of the urine and its appearance, noting whether it is clear or turbid (page 6).

II. Ascertain the specific gravity (page 9).

III. Examine the reaction to litmus paper; and note whether acid, neutral, or alkaline (page 13).

IV. Test the urine for albumen (page 16). If albumen is present look with the microscope for :—

(*a*) Renal Casts (page 94).

(*b*) Pus Corpuscles (page 88).

(*c*) Red Blood Corpuscles (page 45).

V. Test the urine for sugar (page 29).

VI. If the urine be dark coloured test for bile pigments (page 40).

VII. If there be no albumen, nor sugar, nor bile pigment present, and if there be no sediment, the urine need not be further examined, except in special cases.

VIII. If any sediment be observed it must be examined with the microscope (page 67). The following enumeration of the more common deposits may help the student.

 (*a*) Pink, or reddish amorphous deposit, dissolved when a portion of the urine, containing it, is heated in a test-tube. *Urates* (page 72).

 (*b*) Brownish - red crystalline deposit. *Uric Acid* (page 68).

 (*c*) White deposit, crystalline or amorphous, soluble in acetic acid. *Phosphates* (page 78).

 (*d*) Hummocky white sharply defined cloud, insoluble in acetic acid; crystalline. *Oxalate of Lime* (page 75).

 (*e*) White or yellowish flocculent deposit, rendered ropy by addition of liquor potassæ. *Pus* (page 88).

(*f*) White flocculi, amorphous, soluble
in liq. potassæ. *Mucus.*

(*g*) Red non-crystalline deposit, containing red blood corpuscles. *Blood*
(page 87).

PHYSICAL EXAMINATION.

The physical examination of the urine is
the application of the senses to its investigation, with or without the aid of the microscope or other physical instruments, and it
is distinguished from the chemical examination which is its investigation by the aid of
chemical reactions. The quantity, colour,
translucency, odour and consistence are the
chief characters which can be ascertained by
a simple physical examination.

The *quantity* of urine passed daily is about
52 ounces, or 1500 c.c., but it varies within
rather wide limits.

Colour.—Urine is ordinarily of a yellow or
reddish-yellow colour, but it may be as
colourless as water, or red, or dark brown
like porter; the presence of a small quantity
of blood gives it a colour which is well de-

scribed by the word smoky. If bile pigments
are present it may have an orange, or brown,
or dark greenish-brown tint. Many drugs
give a peculiar colour to the urine; *Rhubarb*
and *Senna* colour it reddish-brown, from the
effect of the chrysophanic acid they contain ;
Santonin gives the urine a bright yellow
colour, which is reddened by alkalies. The
absorption of carbolic acid gives it a dark
hue. Tannin given by the mouth renders it
almost colourless.

The urine is pale (1) *in health*, when large
quantities of fluid have been imbibed (*urina
potus*), and (2) *in disease*, in anæmia, in diabetes, in some nervous diseases (*urina spastica*)
and during convalescence from severe illness.
A pale urine contains little colouring matter
and but a small proportion of solid constituents, except in diabetes mellitus, when a
pale urine may contain a large quantity of
grape sugar (page 29). A pale urine is a
sign that the patient is not suffering from
any high degree of pyrexia.

A high coloured urine occurs (1) *in health*,
after food (*urina cibi*), after much exercise
and after free perspiration, (2) *in disease*, in
fevers and most acute disorders, for in these

considerable metamorphosis of the tissues takes place.

It contains much colouring matter and urea in proportion to the water.

A dark urine should be examined for pigment (page 50).

Odour. It is not yet made out to what body the peculiar smell of the urine is due, nor is it of much importance to the clinical student. When the urine loses its natural smell and becomes fœtid and ammoniacal, the change is due to the decomposition of urea into carbonate of ammonia, and to the formation of sulphur compounds ; in cases of cystitis and paraplegia the alteration begins either before or very quickly after the urine has been voided. Certain drugs, as copaiba, and oil of sandal wood, and certain articles of diet, as asparagus, give a characteristic smell to the urine; turpentine gives the odour of violets to the secretion.

If the urine is turbid when first voided it should be carefully examined under the microscope. Pus is a common cause of this appearance, but a slight turbidity is often seen in freshly passed urine, if it be neutral or alkaline, and it is occasioned by the precipitation of phosphates which occurs under such circumstances. Urine which has been retained for some time in the bladder is likely to be slightly turbid from the presence of rather more than the usual quantity of mucus.

Translucency. In health the urine deposits, after remaining at rest for a short time, a slight cloud of mucus, derived from the bladder and urinary passages; but, in all other respects, healthy urine is perfectly clear. On cooling, however, it may sometimes become turbid from the presence of urates, which are distinguished from other deposits by their appearance, upon standing, in urine which was perfectly clear when first passed.

Consistence. The urine is a limpid fluid, flowing freely from one vessel to another. But in catarrh of the bladder and in retention of urine, the ammoniacal products of the decomposition of the urea render the pus present thick and viscid, thus causing the secretion to be ropy, and when this condition is well marked, the urine may be so viscid as to flow with difficulty when poured from one vessel to another.

The froth on normal urine readily disappears ; but if the froth be persistent, the presence of albumen, or of bile pigment, may be suspected.

Before passing to the chemical examination of the urine, it may be well to speak of the apparatus and reagents which will be found necessary by the student for bedside investigation.   They are :—

Cylindrical and Conical Urine Glasses, each containing about 6 fluid-ounces.

A Urinometer, the stem of which is graduated from 1000 to 1060.

Blue and Red Litmus Paper.

Test Tubes.

A Spirit Lamp, or Bunsen's Gas Burner.

Nitric Acid.

Acetic Acid.

Liquor Potassæ or Liquor Sodæ.

Solution of Sulphate of Copper, 10 grains to the fluid-ounce, or Fehling's Test Solution for Sugar (p. 33).

Glass Funnels and Filtering Paper.

With this apparatus and these reagents the student will be able to perform the more important qualitative tests described below.

SPECIFIC GRAVITY.

The specific gravity of a liquid is the number which expresses the relation of the weight of a given volume of the liquid to the weight of the same volume of distilled water.

The specific gravity of the urine varies in health between 1010 and 1035, if the specific gravity of distilled water be taken as 1000. That is to say, a given volume of urine of a specific gravity of 1020 would be heavier than the same volume of distilled water in the proportion of 1020 to 1000.

The simplest way of estimating the specific gravity of the urine is by means of the urinometer (fig. 1). This instrument consists of a hollow glass vessel, weighted below, and terminating above in a slender stem. Its weight is so adjusted that it sinks deeply in distilled water. In denser liquids it sinks less deeply, and less of the stem is submerged; and by means of a suitably graduated scale fixed in the stem, the specific gravity of the urine may be read off directly by observing the number on the scale which

most nearly corresponds to the surface of
the urine.

In order to use this instrument, a quantity
of the urine is poured into a cylindrical glass,

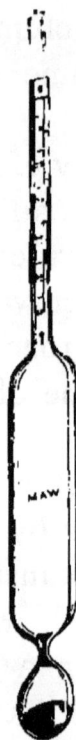

FIG. 1.—Urinometer.

and care must be taken to remove any froth
which may be present; this can be done
with blotting paper, or by overfilling the
vessel. The urinometer must then be care-

fully introduced and allowed to float freely in the urine without touching the side or the bottom of the glass. Since the surface of the fluid rises by capillary attraction round the stem of the instrument, the specific gravity will be too low, if read off with the eye above the level of the liquid; to obtain a correct reading the eye must be lowered to the level of the surface of the fluid, and the number on the stem ascertained by looking at it through the urine.

Having noted this, depress the instrument in the urine, and allow it to come to rest once more, then repeat the reading to verify the first observation. The specific gravity thus ascertained should be noted down at once.

The urine should be at the temperature of the surrounding air; if the specific gravity be taken while the urine is warm, the readings will be too low in about the proportion of one degree of the urinometer for every seven degrees Fahrenheit above the temperature for which the instrument was graduated.

The knowledge of the specific gravity of a few ounces of urine is a matter of little value.

To render the observation in any way serviceable, the whole quantity passed in the 24 hours must be collected and mixed, and the specific gravity of this taken. A rough estimation of the solid matters passed may be made from the specific gravity in the following way ; the two last figures are multiplied by 2 or more correctly, 2·33, and the product gives the amount of solid matters in 1000 parts of urine; if, for example, the specific gravity of the urine be 1020, 1000 grains of urine will contain 20 × 2 = 40 grains of solids, or multiplying by 2·33 = 46·6 grains.

If the quantity of urine is too small to float the urinometer, the specific gravity can be obtained in the following way. Add to the urine one, two, or three times its volume, carefully measured, of distilled water, take the specific gravity of the mixture, and multiply by the number of volumes employed. If three volumes of water were used to dilute one volume of urine, and the specific gravity of this were found to be 1005, then four volumes multiplied by 5 would be 20, and 1020 would be the specific gravity of the urine.

Clinical Import.—A *high* specific gravity may be due to the presence of sugar; if this body is not present, then excess of urea will be the probable cause.

A *low* specific gravity, below 1010, occurs after fluid has been taken in quantity, and in diuresis from any cause, such as exposure to cold, or mental emotion, or after a paroxysm of hysteria. A low specific gravity is also noticed frequently in anæmic states, and it is a common symptom in chronic interstitial nephritis.

A new urinometer should be carefully tested, as they are sometimes carelessly graduated. As a rule the smaller instruments are less correct than the larger ones. A large urinometer and a large amount of urine give the truest results.

REACTION.

If all the urine passed in twenty-four hours by a healthy person be collected and mixed, the reaction of the whole quantity will be acid. The degree of acidity, however, is not uniform, but varies throughout the twenty-four hours, and after a meal the urine may be neutral or alkaline for a time; This has been called the time of "the alkaline tide" by Sir William Roberts; and it is supposed to be associated with the large secretion of acid gastric juice at that time. To neutralize the acidity of the urine passed in twenty-four hours requires about fourteen grains of sodium carbonate.

The acidity of the urine is due to the presence of an acid salt, acid sodium phosphate, NaH_2PO_4, and not to the presence of free acids. It is probable that the organic acids of urine (uric acid, hippuric acid, &c.), are present only in combination with alkaline bases; and therefore they are without influence upon the reaction of normal urine.

The acidity of the urine is said to increase a little during the first few hours after being voided, but sooner or later decomposition sets in, with conversion of the urea into ammonium carbonate and water by the agency of a special ferment, (the *micrococcus ureæ*); the urine then becomes alkaline, and ammoniacal, and fœtid from the presence of ammonium sulphides, while the earthy phosphates, and ammonium urate are deposited as a white sediment.

In many of the cases in which the urine is found to be alkaline, the alkalinity is due to decomposition, taking place after the urine has been passed; therefore if a patient's urine is found to be alkaline, a fresh specimen should be obtained and tested immediately. It is also important to know whether the alkalinity is due to ammonium carbonate or to fixed alkali. When the alkalinity is due to ammonium carbonate, red litmus paper which has been turned blue by the urine will lose its blue colour if gently warmed and dried, but it will remain blue if the alkalinity is due to potash of soda.

When urine owes its alkalinity to ammonium carbonate, it is almost certainly due to decomposition of the urea; this decomposition takes place in the bladder itself in cases of cystitis, in paraplegia, and in retention of urine, if by any means the *micrococcus ureæ* has gained an entry into the bladder, as frequently happens after the use of sounds or catheters which have previously been in contact with urine undergoing the ammoniacal fermentation. In health the urine can be made alkaline by medicines which contain the fixed alkalies either in the form of hydrates, carbonates, or alkaline phosphates, or in combination with most organic acids such as acetates, citrates, tartrates, in which cases the alkali is excreted as an alkaline carbonate. The administration of ammonia either free or combined does not make the urine alkaline. A diet consisting largely of meat tends to increase the acidity of the urine, and a vegetarian diet tends to make the urine alkaline. It is not so easy to make the urine acid by the administration of drugs as it is to make it alkaline, but the mineral acids do increase the acidity of the urine to a certain extent; and there are certain organic acids which are excreted as acids, and tend to increase the acidity of the urine. Benzoic acid, which is excreted as Hippuric acid, is one of the best known instances.

The acidity of urine is increased by fasting, and is apparently increased when the urinary water is diminished, and the urine thereby rendered more concentrated.

EXAMINATION FOR ALBUMEN.

This is the first and most important step in the chemical examination of the urine:

the presence or absence of albumen must always be determined before proceeding to test for any other substance, and the search must never be omitted in the examination of any urine.

A very large number of reagents have been proposed as tests for albumen in the urine. They all act by coagulation and precipitation of the albumen, which is thus rendered visible. It will be sufficient to describe three methods of testing for albumen, viz :—

(1) Coagulation by heat and acid.

(2) Coagulation by concentrated nitric acid in the cold. (Heller's test).

(3) Coagulation by picric acid.

(1) *By heat and acid.*—The best way of performing this test is to fill a test tube about two-thirds full of the urine to be examined, and to heat the upper layers of the fluid over the flame of a lamp, the lower part of the tube being held between the thumb and forefinger of the observer, in the manner represented in the following woodcut (fig. 2). By employing this method of procedure, the boiled upper part of the urine can be compared with the unboiled portion in the lower

part of the tube, and any slight degree
of turbidity produced by the boiling can
be readily perceived.   It is a very useful
precaution to filter the urine before boiling
it; this step is too commonly neglected, but
when the urine is a all turbid it should
always be filtered before testing for albumen,
for it is very much easier to see any faint

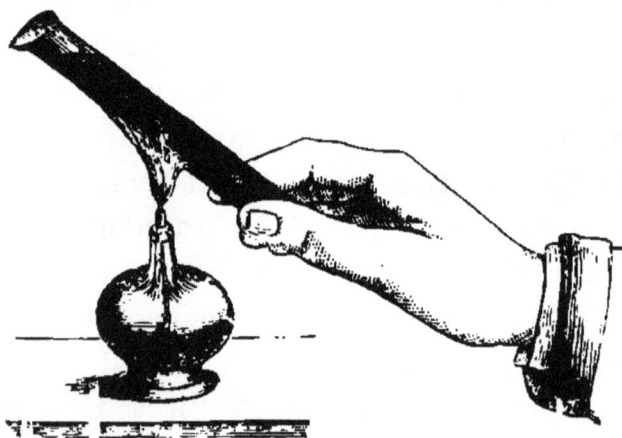

Fig. 2.

cloud of turbidity produced by the test if the
urine under examination is first rendered
perfectly bright and clear.   The heat must be
applied until the upper portion of the urine
boils, and it is as well to keep it boiling for a
full minute, otherwise, in certain cases, scme
of the albumen may escape coagulation.   The

boiled layer of fluid should now be carefully compared with the cool layer in the lower part of the tube, by holding the test tube in a good light, and looking through it at a dark background, for example, the sleeve of one's coat. If any cloudiness or turbidity be seen, it must not at once be concluded that albumen is present ; a drop or two of acetic acid or nitric acid should first be added. The cloud is permanent if due to albumen, but disappears quickly if due to phosphates. This addition of acid after boiling should never be omitted, since the most practised eye cannot distinguish, by appearance only, between the cloud of albumen, and the cloud of phosphate of lime.

Cautions. The nitric acid must be added carefully, and not more than two drops used, otherwise the coagulated albumen if present only in small quantity may be redissolved, and the urine may be wrongly thought to be free from albumen. It is much better to acidify with strong acetic acid, and not to use nitric acid for this test at all.

The effervescence which is often noticed, when nitric acid is added to the urine, is due to the decomposition of the urea by the

nitrous acid which is so commonly present
as an impurity. The gases evolved are
carbon dioxide and nitrogen. • Should the
urine be turbid from the presence of urates,
it may be made clear by gently warming the
contents of the test tube before boiling the
upper layers. It is often more convenient to
clear such urines by gentle heat rather than
by filtration.

If the urine be neutral or alkaline at the
time of testing, it may be carefully acidified
by a few drops of dilute acetic acid before
boiling ; but it is better not to do so, lest the
albumen be converted into acid albumen,
and give no precipitate on boiling. If the
preliminary acidification be done with nitric
or hydrochloric acids this change into acid
albumen is almost certain to be the result.

If the urine be alkaline the albumen may
be present as alkali-albumen; and this body
also gives no precipitate on boiling alone but
this is not likely to mislead because the precipitate will appear as soon as the drop or
two of strong acid is added after the boiling.

The precipitate of phosphate of lime
which is produced when certain urines are
boiled always disappears when the acid is

added. This precipitate is not a sign that
the urine under examination is rich in phosphates, but signifies rather that the specimen is deficient in acidity.

(2) *Precipitation by concentrated nitric acid
without heat. Heller's test.*

The addition of strong nitric acid to albuminous urine will usually coagulate the
albumen; the most delicate mode of applying the test is by the method proposed by
Heller, which consists in pouring some
strong nitric acid into a test-tube, and
afterwards adding the urine to be tested, in
such a way as to avoid mixing the two
fluids; this is done by holding the test-tube
in a very much inclined position and allowing the urine to flow in very gently along
the side of the tube. When this operation is
carefully carried out the two fluids touch
but do not mix, the nitric acid, owing to
its greater density, remaining in the lower
stratum. If albumen be present a whitish
ring or disc of coagulated albumen gradually
forms at the line of contact of the two liquids.
Unless the urine is quite clear and bright,
the test is not very delicate; but it is easy to
filter the urine and indeed the neatest way of

bringing the two liquids into contact, un-
mixed, is to let the urine flow down the side
of the test-tube from the filter itself.

Heller's test is thought highly of by many
people, but it is not so good a test as the
one by heat and acetic acid. Urea nitrate
may form in concentrated urines, and mislead, and uric acid may do the same.

Copaiba taken internally causes a precipitate to appear in the urine with nitric
acid in the cold, and so imitates the coagulation of albumen. It does not give any
reaction with heat and acetic acid.

(3) *The picric acid test.* A saturated solution of picric acid coagulates albumen in
neutral or acid urine; it is usually recommended to acidify the urine with citric acid
before applying the test, but this is rarely
necessary, the picric acid itself will generally
be sufficient to ensure that the mixture shall
not be alkaline.

To carry out the test, fill a test-tube half
full of the urine, filtered if necessary, and
then pour upon it picric acid solution to the
depth of about an inch, if albumen is present
a white cloud will be formed at the junction
of the two fluids, and may be increased by

gently shaking the tube so that the fluids mix near their point of junction.

The compound of picric acid and albumen is soluble in excess of albumen, but this is not a serious objection to its use in testing urines, as it can easily be guarded against by a little care and attention.

(4) *Potassio-mercuric iodide (Tanret's test)*[*] is also recommended as a good test for albumen. It is extremely delicate, indeed, perhaps too much so, for it is said to produce a slight opalescence in al urines.

Among other suggested tests for albumen in the urine may be mentioned tungstate of soda and ferrocyanide of potassium (both of these must be applied to urines which have previously been acidified with acetic or citric acid) and Sir William Roberts' acidulated brine test (saturated solution of sodium chloride 19 parts, strong hydrochloric acid 1 part). A paper by Dr. Vincent Harris, in vol. xix. of the St. Bartholomew's Hospital Reports should be consulted for full information on these reagents.

To make the testing of urines more con-

---

[*] Mercuric chloride 1·35 grammes, potassium iodide 3·32 grammes, acetic acid 20 c.c., water 64 c.c.

venient for practitioners Dr. Oliver[*] of Harrogate has contrived a series of test papers charged with the proper reagents by means of which albumen may be readily discovered in the urine, and he has extended the same methods to the testing for sugar, bile pigment and bile salts.

The ordinary prcteids occurring in the urine are (1) *serum-albumen*, (2) *paraglobulin;* both of these bodies are present in ordinary cases of albuminuria, though their relative proportions may vary a good deal (3) *acid albumen*, and *alkali albumen* may also occur, but their presence is due to changes in the urine after its secretion by the kidney, (4) *albumoses* and *peptone* may also be found; perhaps most of the cases reported as peptonuria should be regarded as cases of urine containing albumose.

The presence of these bodies may be ascertained by the biuret test; the urine is first made alkaline with liquor potassæ, and then a drop of a dilute solution of sulphate of copper is added and the mixture is well shaken. A rose colour appears if albumose or peptone be present.

[*] On Bed-side Urine Testing. By Dr. Geo. Oliver. H. K. Lewis.

This test can, however, but seldom be applied directly to the urine; if other albuminous bodies be present it is absolutely necessary that they be removed; and if the urine be high coloured, it will be necessary to decolorise it with carbonate of lead. These more elaborate processes can seldom be employed by the clinical clerk.*

Albumoses have been found in the urine in such conditions as scurvy, purpura, and other acute hæmorrhagic diseases; also in those cases where a large number of white corpuscles are being destroyed, as in the absorption of large pleuritic effusions, in pneumonia, inflammation of the joints, meningitis, fractures, boils, &c.

A rough way of estimating the amount of albumen present in the urine, is to pour some of the urine into a test-tube, until it be about half full, and to boil the whole of the urine in the tube, till the albumen be completely coagulated. One or two drops of nitric acid are then added and the test-tube is set aside

---

* See Textbook of Chemical Physiology and Pathology, Dr. Halliburton. *Longmans & Co.* "The detection of proteid bodies in the urine," Dr. Sydney Martin. *Brit. Med. Jour.*, April, 1888.

for twenty-four hours; at the end of that time the proportion of the coagulated albumen which has collected at the bottom of the tube, to the rest of the fluid is noticed: if the albumen occupy one-third of the height of the fluid there is said to be one-third of albumen in the urine, and so for one-sixth, or one-eighth, as may be. If, however, at the end of 24 hours scarcely any albumen have collected at the bottom, there is said to be a trace. If any urates have been deposited, the urine must be filtered before boiling, or a considerable error will creep in, by their increasing the apparent amount of albumen.

This method of estimating the albumen quantitatively has been elaborated by the use of graduated test-tubes. Esbach's "albuminometer" (fig. 3) is such a tube; to use it, urine is poured in to reach the graduation U. and saturated picric acid solution is added to the mark R, the tube is shaken and the fluids mixed, the coagulated albumen is then left to settle for twenty-four hours and the number opposite to its upper level at the end of that time is read off directly as grammes per litre of dry albumen. To express the result as a percentage divide by 10 because a litre of water weighs 1000 grammes.

Clinical import.—The presence of albumen in the urine is an important objective sign of

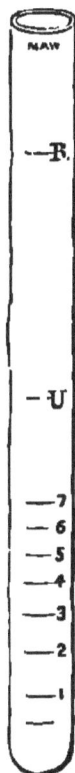

Fig. 3.—Esbach's Albuminometer.

disease.   The causes of albuminuria may be grouped under the following heads :—

(1) Obstruction to the flow of blood through the kidneys.

Any state which brings about a mechanical impediment to the return of blood from the kidneys, will be accompanied by albumen in the urine, and the albumen will be persistent so long as the congestion of the kidney continues ; the longer the state of congestion remains, the greater danger is there of permanent textural injury to the kidney. Any *general* impediment to the circulation, such as valvular disease of the heart, or emphysema of the lungs, or any *local* impediment to the renal circulation, as from a tumour pressing upon the renal veins or inferior *vena cava*, will produce albuminuria.

(2) Any acute febrile disease may be accompanied by albuminuria, which, as a rule, disappears with the disappearance of the febrile state, unless there be some permanent structural change set up thereby in the kidney.

(3) Diseases of the kidney itself are usually accompanied by albuminuria.

It must not be forgotten that albumen may find its way with the urine from any part of the urinary tract, from the ureters, as when they are lacerated by the passage of a calculus; from the bladder, in many diseased conditions of that viscus ; from the urethra in gonorrhœa, or from the vagina. In the urine of women, a small quantity of albumen is often due to leucorrhœal discharge, which is composed partly of pus.

If blood be present in the urine, albumen must likewise be present, derived from the corpuscles and plasma.

The search for renal casts (p. 94) must always follow the detection of albumen in the urine. The discovery of these structures renders it certain that the albumen, or at least part of it, is derived from the kidney.

EXAMINATION FOR SUGAR.

If the specific gravity rise above 1030, sugar may be suspected, and should be looked for. Sugar may also occur in urines of low specific gravity.

The sugar in the urine is grape sugar.

Many methods of testing for sugar have been proposed ; but only the most prominent and trustworthy will here be mentioned.

Before testing urine for sugar, it should be

tested for *albumen;* and if this body be
present, it should be removed by boiling
and acidulating some of the urine with one
or two drops of acetic acid, and filtering. In
the same way if the urine be high coloured,
it may be well to get rid of the colouring
matters by throwing them down with a solution of acetate of lead and filtering. And if
the urine be turbid from urates, it is very
desirable to free the urine from these by filtration before applying the tests for sugar.

Moore's test.—Equal parts of urine, and
liquor potassæ or liquor sodæ, are poured
into a test tube, and the upper layer of this
mixture is heated to boiling, in the manner
described in the section on examination for
albumen. (See p. 17). The heated portion
becomes brown or dark brown, according to
the quantity of sugar present. The least
change of colour may be perceived by com-
paring the upper and lower layers of the
liquid.

Caution.—High-coloured urines and indeed
almost all urines darken very perceptibly on
boiling with caustic alkalies, and if the urine
be albuminous, the colour will be greatly
deepened, though no sugar be present. This

test, therefore, is not worthy of the attention of a careful student.

The Copper test depends on the property which grape sugar possesses, of reducing the higher oxide of copper (CuO) to a suboxide (Cu_2O). There are two methods of conducting this reaction, identical in principle, named respectively Trommer's Test and Fehling's Test.

Trommer's test.—About a drachm of the suspected urine is poured into a test tube, and liquor potassæ or liquor sodæ added in about the same quantity : a weak solution of sulphate of copper (about 10 grains to the fluid ounce) is dropped into the mixture. If sugar is present the precipitate which first forms is redissolved on shaking the test tube, and the copper solution should be carefully added, shaking the test tube after each drop has fallen into the mixture, so long as the precipitate is easily redissolved, when the solution will have acquired a beautiful blue colour, but should be quite clear, and free from any blue precipitate ; the contents of the test tube must next be heated to boiling, when, if, sugar be present, an orange red precipitate is first thrown down, which, after

some time, becomes reddish brown. This
precipitate consists of the suboxide of copper
or cuprous oxide.

On applying Trommer's test to urine, a
change of colour is seen in every case; but
this is no proof of the presence of sugar ; the
reaction is only known to be complete when
a red or orange precipitate is thrown down.

If the test be carefully done with urine
which contains no sugar, or other reducing
substances, the following points will be
noticed:—1. The mixture is of a pale blue or
green colour, and not of the deep blue which
is seen when sugar is present.   2. The flocculent precipitate of cupric hydrate is not
redissolved, even though it may seem to be,
and if the mixture be filtered it will come
through without any blue tinge.   3. Boiling
produces a yellowish colouration of the mixture from the action of the excess of alkali
upon the colouring matters of the urine, (see
Moore's test above), and floating in the mixture may be seen flakes of phosphate of lime,
thrown down by the potash, and black particles of cupric oxide the result of the decomposition of the cupric hydrate by the heat
employed.

When sugar is present, the cupric hydrate redissolves to form a rich deep blue solution, which will pass through the filter, and boiling throws down àn opaque precipitate of the red cuprous oxide.

Since uric acid and mucus will also reduce copper when they are boiled with its salts in an alkaline solution the test should be tried also in the cold, and if at the end of the twenty-four hours the reddish precipitate have fallen, sugar is undoubtedly present.

Cautions.—Much trouble is often at first felt in arranging the proper proportion between the copper solution, and the liquor potassæ. The mixture must be alkaline, too much copper must not be added ; and it is wise, in every doubtful case, to filter, and operate with a clear solution.

Fehling's solution. (Dr. Pavy's solution is identical in principle with Fehling's solution). In consequence of the difficulty of properly adjusting the quantity of alkali and copper in Trommer's test, many practitioners prefer to use a solution in which the copper and alkali are present in the exact proportion necessary. This solution may be prepared in the following way :—665½ grains of crystallized

potassio-tartrate of soda are dissolved in 5
fluid ounces of a solution of caustic potash, sp.
gr. 1·12. Into this alkaline solution is poured
a fluid prepared by dissolving 133½ grains of
sulphate of copper in 10 fluid drachms of
water. The solution is exceedingly apt to
decompose, and must always be kept in
stoppered bottles, and in a cool place. It
is usually, therefore, more convenient not to
mix the alkali and copper until the solution
is wanted for use. In this case, a fluid
drachm of the sulphate of copper solution may
be added to half a fluid ounce of the alkaline
solution of potassio-tartrate of soda prepared
as above.

About a couple of drachms of this test-
solution are poured into an ordinary test-
tube, and the fluid boiled over a lamp. If
no deposit form, the solution may be used
for analysis; but if a red precipitate be
thrown down, the liquid has decomposed,
and a fresh supply must be had.

While the solution is boiling in the test-
tube, the urine must be added to it, drop by
drop, and the effect watched. A few drops
of urine which contain a large percentage of
sugar will at once give a precipitate of yel-

low or red suboxide; but if no precipitate occur, the urine should be added to the fluid drop by drop, any deposit being carefully looked for, until a quantity equal to that of the Fehling's solution employed has been added. If no precipitate be found after setting the test-tube aside for an hour, the urine may be considered free from sugar.

Cautions.—1. The test solution should never be used without boiling beforehand for a few seconds; for the tartrate is exceedingly apt to decompose, and the solution then reduces itself as effectually as if grape sugar were present.

2. The quantity of urine used in the test should never be greater than the quantity of test solution employed.

3. After adding urine in volume equal to the Fehling's solution, the boiling of the mixture must not be continued, as other bodies present in the urine, besides sugar, may reduce copper at a prolonged high temperature.

Fermentation test.—Two portions of the urine are taken, and put into two flasks; to one a few grains of German yeast is added; both are then set aside in a warm place. Fermentation sets in in that flask to which the yeast has been added, and the sugar is thereby split up into alcohol and carbon dioxide, and from the loss of weight which results, the quantity of sugar present can be calculated.

Estimation by loss of density after fermentation. Sir William Roberts has shown, that, after fermentation, " the number of degrees of ' density lost ' indicated as many grains of sugar per fluid ounce," and he proposes to estimate by this means the amount of sugar present.

In twenty-four hours the fermentation is almost finished ; the fermented urine is poured into a urine glass, and the specific gravity taken with the urinometer ; the specific gravity of the unfermented urine is also taken, and the specific gravity of the fermented is subtracted from the specific gravity of the unfermented, the remainder giving the number of grains of sugar contained in a fluid ounce ; for example, if the specific gravity of the unfermented be 1040, and that of the fermented 1010, the number of grains of sugar in a fluid ounce will be 30.

Indigo-carmine test.—When indigo-blue or indigo-carmine (sulphindigotate or soda) is heated with an alkali in the presence of glucose, it loses its colour and becomes indigo-white, which when oxidised becomes indigo-blue again. Dr. Oliver has taken advantage of this reaction to contrive a test for sugar, and has prepared a test paper upon which indigo-carmine has been deposited : the paper is introduced with some carbonate of soda into a test-tube ; enough distilled or common water is poured into the tube to cover the papers and heat applied; the solution thus prepared should be of a fine blue colour. To the blue solution a drop or two of the suspected urine may now be added, and the contents of the test-tube again warmed, but not boiled or shaken ; if sugar be present, the blue colour of the indigo is quickly discharged, and the solution becomes yellow ; if the solution be now cooled and shaken, blue streaks pass down into the fluid from the surface, and if the shaking be continued, the fluid becomes of its original blue colour, and may again be decolourised by again warming it.

The picric acid test.—Equal parts of liquor potassæ and saturated solution of picric acid are mixed, and boiled in a test-tube. The

mixture is then divided into two equal parts,
in two similar test-tubes.   A little of the suspected urine is added to one of them, and
both are again boiled for a few moments.   If
sugar is present a deep brown colour will be
developed in the one tube.   The other is
needed for purposes of comparison, because
some darkening of colour is always produced
when the mixture is boiled, whether sugar be
present or not.

Phenyl-hydrazine test.—Add to the urine a
little acetate of soda, and some phenyl-hydrazine hydrochlorate solution.   Heat in a water
bath to 100° C. for half an hour.   If sugar
be present a yellow crystalline precipitate is
thrown down.

It has been thought that the coma so often
seen at the end of diabetes, is due to the
presence of acetone in the blood, and the
state has been named acetonæmia.   The
urine will then often give a deep red reaction
with perchloride of iron, a reaction which is
thought to be due to the presence of acetone,
acetonuria.   Dr. Ralfe tests for the presence
of acetone in the urine in the following way :—
a drachm of liquor potassæ in which about
twenty grains of iodide of potassium have

been dissolved is boiled in a test-tube : while still hot, a drachm of the urine to be tested is poured on to the surface of the fluid, as in Heller's test (see p. 21) and at the line of contact, a ring of phosphate appears ; and if acetone be present, the colour of the ring becomes in a few minutes yellow, and numerous yellow points of iodoform appear, which later on sink to the bottom of the test-tube.

It is still disputed whether the urine in health contain sugar. Brücke holds that a healthy man excretes daily through the kidneys about fifteen grains of sugar. According to Leube, the excretion of sugar in diabetes is far greater during the night, than during the day: urea follows just the opposite rule.

Clinical Import.—If the foregoing tests announce the presence of sugar, in considerable quantity, as often as the urine is examined, diabetes mellitus may be inferred to exist. But should the presence of sugar in the urine be variable, and amount small, the fact is not of any known great diagnostic or therapeutic importance.

Sugar is said to be present in the urine of

the fœtus; of women when suckling, and of some old persons. It is seen in the urine during convalescence from some acute disorders, especially cholera, in malarious diseases, and in carbuncle. Certain injuries of the nervous system also bring on glycosuria.

BILE IN THE URINE.

The presence of bile in the urine can seldom be overlooked, since it gives a dark orange or greenish brown colour to the secretion. White filtering paper is coloured yellow by the urine; a permanent froth is also formed by shaking the urine. The colour given to the urine by drugs such as rhubarb and santonin is distinguished from that given by the bile pigments by the reaction of alkalies. Alkalies deepen the red of vegetable pigments, but turn bilious urine to a dirty brown.

Two bodies must be tested for, the bile pigments and the bile acids, each of which must be looked for by itself.

THE BILE PIGMENTS.—*Gmelin's test.*—Ordinary nitric acid, which is slightly yellow and contains some nitrous acid, is poured into a test-tube to the depth of half an inch. A portion of the urine to be examined is then gently poured down the side of the tube, held almost horizontally, on to the surface of the acid, so that the two fluids may touch but not mix ; this operation is most conveniently performed by means of a pipette. The test-tube may then be nearly filled with urine. At the line of contact, a zone of red appears in every urine; but if bile pigment be present, the layer of urine above becomes green. This is the characteristic colour ; without the green colour the presence of bile pigments cannot be predicated. This reaction may also be performed by allowing a drop of nitric acid and one of the urine to run together on a porcelain dish, when a play of colours with green will be observed at the line of contact. But this is not so good as the first method, as the green colour is less perfectly seen. By waiting a few minutes, the green colour will sometimes develop in a fluid which at first gave no reaction.

Caution.—Any urine which contains a large amount of colouring matter will give a red-dish or purple colour with nitric acid. The green colour, however, is not seen with any other body than bile pigment.

Iodine test.—Some solution of iodine, not more than a drop or two, should be added to the urine in a test-tube, and if bile pigment be present, the whole becomes of a fine green colour. The green colour is perhaps due to the formation of the same body, biliverdin, which causes the green reaction in Gmelin's test.

THE BILE SALTS.—*Pettenkofer's test.*—This test depends upon the reaction given by the bile acids with sulphuric acid and cane sugar, to produce a purple colour.

Pettenkofer's test should never be applied directly to urine: the bile acids are never present in sufficient quantity to give the reaction, however modified, and the urine in jaundice frequently contains a small quantity of albumen which gives a reddish violet reaction with sugar and sulphuric acid, while the action of the acid upon the other coloured constituents of the urine renders it impossible to be sure of the distinctive colours of Pettenkofer's test. If, therefore, it be very desirable to ascertain whether the bile acids be present in the urine, the following method must be employed for their separation ; a long and somewhat complicated process, which can seldom be adopted by the clinical student.

Mix several ounces of the urine with animal charcoal to form a soft paste, and evaporate to dryness over a water bath, stirring the mixture from time to time; when quite dry, extract with hot absolute alcohol ; concentrate, and apply Pettenkofer's test as follows :—To a portion of the concentrated alcoholic extract in a porcelain dish add a drop of cane sugar syrup, mix well with a glass rod, add one drop of strong sulphuric acid, mix again, and warm very gently and gradually. A purple colour develops if bile salts are present.

Hay's test.—Urine containing bile salts has a lower surface tension than that of urine in which no bile salts are present, and for that reason finely powdered sulphur, which will float on the surface of water, will sink rapidly in urine to which a trace of bile salt has been added.

If this test be applied to urine it will be found that the sulphur falls more readily through the surface of any urine than through distilled water, and through the surface of urine containing bile salts more readily still.

A solution of commercial peptone has also been made use of by Dr. Oliver for the detection of bile salts in the urine; and conversely, a solution of bile salts may be used for the detection of peptonuria. The precipitation is, according to Dr. Halliburton, a reaction between the bile salts and albumose; true peptone not being precipitated by bile salts.

BLOOD.

Blood is not at all infrequently found in the urine, and it may be derived from any part of the urinary tract. If derived from the kidneys, the blood will be completely diffused through the urine, and give it a peculiar smoky appearance, quite diagnostic. If the hæmorrhage from the kidney be great the urine will have a bright red colour, like blood; and there may be a distinct sediment of red blood corpuscles at the bottom of the urine glass.

The microscopic test.—In any case where the

presence of blood is suspected the urine
must be examined under the microscope for
red blood corpuscles; as these tend to settle
to the bottom, a drop of the fluid should be
taken up with a pipette from the lowest part
of the vessel, the corpuscles if present will
then be readily seen, unless the sample of
urine be a stale one.

Their peculiar shape and colour will pre-

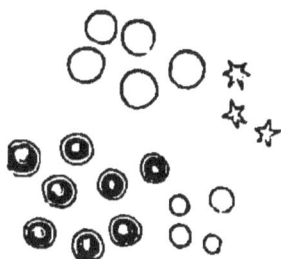

Fig. 4.—Blood corpuscles in the urine.

vent the student mistaking them for any
other deposit; they may, however, in a
urine of low specific gravity, become swollen,
pale, and at last burst from endosmosis; in
those of high specific gravity, they will often
become contracted, shrivelled and distorted,
from exosmosis.

The urine will, of course, contain albumen
in proportion to the quantity of blood present, which may be so great that the urine

will solidify on the application of heat. The urine readily becomes alkaline, and steps may be taken to restore the acid reaction with acetic acid, before testing for albumen.

The spectroscope test.—As part of the hæmoglobin passes from the corpuscles and is held in solution in the urine, it is as well also to examine this with the spectroscope, when the characteristic absorption bands of hæmoglobin will be seen, usually in the form of oxyhæmoglobin.

In some cases the hæmoglobin may be partly or wholly converted into methæmoglobin, especially when the urine has become stale before it is examined. And also in cases of poisoning by chlorate of potassium the same body has been found in the urine.

The guaiacum test.—A few drops of the tincture of guaiacum are added to the urine in a test tube, and then an excess of ozonic ether, that is a mixture of peroxide of hydrogen and ether. The mixture is shaken together, and on standing, the ether separates; of a fine sapphire blue colour, if blood be present.

The reaction depends upon the oxidation of the guaiacum by the ozonic ether; this

however, it is unable to do save in the presence of a body like hæmoglobin; so that it
is the presence of the hæmoglobin which de-
termines the reaction.

The results of this test must always be
received with caution, and can hardly be
accepted unless confirmed by other evidence.
Many other bodies besides hæmoglobin seem
able to determine the oxidation of the
guaiacum.

The hæmin test.—The formation of hæmin
crystals can also be applied as a test for
blood in the urine, but it is more adapted to
the detection of blood in urinary sediment,
and will be considered under that heading
(p. 87). Hæmatoporphyrin also occurs in
urine and will be dealt with in the next
section on urinary pigments.

Clinical import.—The presence of blood, or
of blood corpuscles, in the urine is a sign of
hæmorrhage from the kidney or the urinary
passages. It may result from :—

    1. *Disease of the Kidney.*
        Acute or Chronic Nephritis.
        Congestion of kidney.
        Cancer of kidney.
        External injury.

2. *Disease of Renal Pelvis and Ureter.*
   Calculus.
   Parasite, as Bilharzia hæmatobia.
   Cancer.
3. *Disease of the Bladder.*
   Calculus.
   Cancerous or villous growths.
   Congestion or ulceration of mucous
      membrane.
4. *Disease of the Urethra.*
   Congestion, as in gonorrhœa.
   Tearing of the mucous membrane
      from mechanical injury.
5. In women, uterine discharges, as
   menstruation, &c.

If the amount of blood in the urine be
small, the chances favour the belief that the
blood is derived from the kidneys; search
must therefore be made for renal casts. If
the amount of blood be large, it probably
comes from the pelvis of the kidney, ureter,
or bladder; if from the pelvis or ureter, there
may be pus, and possibly also gravel in the
urine, with pains in the loins, passing down
into the thighs and testicles. If there be
none of these indications, the blood probably
comes from the bladder. It is commonly

said, that if the blood be completely mixed with the urine, the hæmorrhage is from the kidneys; if the urine first passed be clear, and that at the end of micturition become bloody, or if even pure blood be passed, the hæmorrhage is from the bladder or prostate; while if the first portion of the urine be bloody, and the last drops clear, the hæmorrhage is from the urethra. These rules will, however, often be found to fail.

In certain other diseases it is said that hæmoglobin may be detected by chemical tests, but yet no blood corpuscles seen with the microscope; such as poisoning by arsen-iuretted hydrogen, phosphorus, and sulphuric acid; in jaundice, malignant cases of the acute specific diseases, and scurvy. Also in the disease called paroxysmal hæmaturia, it is said that no corpuscles can be found.

One of the chief dangers of hæmaturia is the formation of clots in the passages, and consequent ischuria. Small clots may sometimes form the nucleus of a calculus.

THE PIGMENTS OF THE URINE.

Our knowledge of the colouring matters of urine is still very imperfect ; the following statement of what is known will suffice for the purposes of this book.

(1) *Urochrome.*—This name has been given to a yellow body, which is the cause of the yellow colour of normal urine ; it is an unstable, non-crystalline body, insoluble in chloroform, and has no special spectroscopic absorption band. It is always present.

(2) *Urobilin.*—This is a red body, soluble in chloroform, which is found in febrile urines, and is in part the cause of their having a red tinge ; it is fluorescent, and gives even in very dilute solutions a dark absorption band near the junction of green and blue of the spectrum.

(3) *Uroerythrin.*—This is the name given to a body which is carried down from certain urines in combination with the urates, and gives them the pink colour which they sometimes present. Urines holding it in solution have an orange-red colour, and usually contain urobilin as well. Its composition is

unknown; in strong alcoholic solution it presents two faint absorption bands in the green part of the spectrum.

Hæmatoporphyrin.—Occasionally one meets with urines of a deep wine-red colour, which give very strongly the spectra of hæmatoporphyrin. Dr. Archibald Garrod has lately shown that traces of hæmatoporphyrin are extremely common in the urine both in health and in disease, and that it is very frequently present in fair amount without producing any special coloration in the urine. In a paper in the *Journal of Physiology*, 1892, p. 598, *et seq.*, he describes methods for extracting the hæmatoporphyrin in a pure form, by means of the process employed by Heller for the precipitation of blood pigments from urine. Liq. potassæ is added to the urine to throw down the earthy phosphates; these carry down the hæmatoporphyrin. After washing with distilled water on a filter the hæmatoporphyrin can be dissolved out of the phosphates by alcohol acidulated with dilute sulphuric acid. In certain febrile states this body is often present in considerable amount, although but seldom in such large quantities as to give

the urine a dark red colour. It is identical
with hæmatoporphyrin prepared artificially
from the blood.

Indigo.—In rare cases an urine of a green
colour containing free indigo blue has been
passed, and it is possible by chemical methods to obtain indigo from many urines.

The name of Indican has been applied to
the urinary body whose decomposition yields
indigo, and urines are said to give the
indican reaction when they yield purple
colours on treatment with strong acids ; a
better name for the indigo producing body is
indoxyl-sulphuric acid, which exists, combined with bases (potash or soda) in most
urines. To test for this body the urine must
be mixed with half its bulk of hydrochloric
acid, and left exposed to the air for twelve
hours, at the end of that time a pellicle of
blue indigo may be found floating on its
surface. This can be filtered off and the
filter dried and treated with warm chloroform, which dissolves the indigo and acquires
a blue colour ; other methods for obtaining
the indigo are to be found in the textbooks
of physiological chemistry. Another body
closely allied to indoxyl-sulphuric acid,

namely skatoxyl-sulphuric acid (skatol is methyl-indol) also occurs in the urine, its presence is the cause of a peculiar pink colour which is sometimes noticed when strong nitric acid is added to certain pale coloured urines.

Melanin.—The urine of patients with melanotic cancer is sometimes of a dark brown colour from the presence of a pigment called melanin. Its history is unknown.

Clinical Import.—Our knowledge of the urinary pigments in health is in so imperfect a state that nothing is known of the changes which they undergo in disease.

In obstruction, catarrh, and other diseases of the small intestines, it is said that there is an increase of indican in the urine.

Cautions.—It is necessary to be on one's guard against certain colour appearances due to drugs. The addition of nitric acid to the urine of a patient taking iodides or bromides causes the development of a brown colour from the liberated iodine or bromine. Fuchsine and certain other of the aniline colours are excreted by the urine, to which they communicate their colour, as also do rhubarb, senna, and santonin.

UREA.

Urea is the body characteristic of the urine; unless a fluid contain urea, it cannot be said to be urine.

The clinical student may sometimes wish to know if the urine contain urea, or if a given fluid be really urine, or some other secretion. The fluid is first to be tested for albumen, which, if present, must be removed by boiling and acidifying with a few drops of acetic acid, and filtering. The filtrate is to be used for the subsequent operation as stated below.

If the urine be free from albumen, some quantity, two or three fluid ounces, must be evaporated in a porcelain dish over a water bath, until the fluid have the consistence of syrup. A water bath is essential, because an open flame would decompose the urea. After the fluid is completely cooled, a drop - may be let fall on a slide, and a drop of strong pure nitric acid may be added with a glass rod.

If the nitric acid be yellow from the presence of nitrous acid, it is unsuitable, as it will oxidise and destroy the urea, but if it be pure then crystals of nitrate of urea will form in flat rhombic or hexagonal plates which may be recognised under the microscope (fig. 5, *b*).

By adding a drop of saturated solution of oxalic acid instead of the nitric acid, crystals

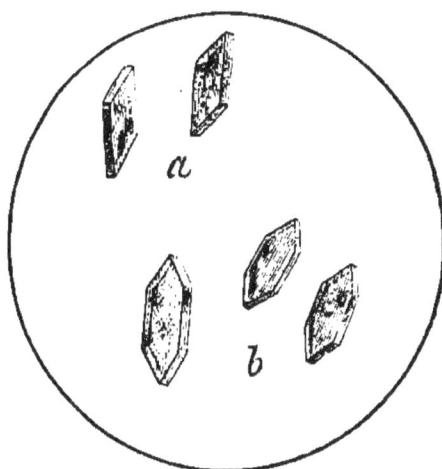

FIG. 5.
a. Oxalate of Urea. *b.* Nitrate of Urea.

of oxalate of urea of somewhat similar shapes will be obtained (fig. 5, *a*).

Sometimes only a few drops of the fluid can be had, and the student should then let a little fall on the glass slide, set it aside in a warm place, protected from dust, for the fluid to concentrate, then add the strong nitric acid, and place the slide under the microscope.

Another simple method of determining the presence of urea in a liquid is to add a little sodium hypobromite or hypochlorite solution. If urea be present, a brisk effervescence is produced. As the reagent gives an effervescence with ammonia it must first be ascertained that ammonia is not present in the liquid.

Clinical Import.—Healthy urine may be looked upon as being for the most part a solution of urea and chloride of sodium; one half of the solids being made up of urea, and one quarter of chloride of sodium. Urea is the most important constituent of the urine; a healthy man excretes from 300 to 500 grains in twenty-four hours. Its amount is increased in health by a free meat diet, and decreased by purely vegetable food. In some acute diseases, as pneumonia, typhoid fever, and acute rheumatism, the urea is greatly increased owing to the excessive tissue-metamorphosis; it may be present in such quantity as to give a mass of crystals, with out previous concentration, when the urine is acidulated with nitric acid. In chronic

diseases, especially those attended by a ca-
chexia, or in uræmia and chronic Bright's
disease, the amount of urea is below the
average. In diabetes, the amount of urea
secreted in twenty-four hours is increased;
although the amount *per cent.* in the urine is
much decreased by the excessive flow of
water which passes out through the kidneys.

URIC ACID.

Uric acid exists in the urine chiefly in the
form of urates of the alkaline metals, potassium and sodium. The average daily quantity excreted is from 7 to 9 grains.

Uric acid is very insoluble in water, re-
quiring 15,000 times its weight of cold water,
and 1,900 times its weight of hot water to
dissolve it. The urates are much less insoluble, but they too are frequently precipitated from solution as the urine becomes cold
on standing.

On this account uric acid, and urates both
form common urinary sediments, and will be
considered under that section.

Usually the uric acid is not free when the

urine is voided, but it is thrown down by the increase of acidity which always occurs shortly after emission. This is especially the case in the urine of diabetes, where the whole of the uric acid present may be set free from this cause.

Uric acid is sometimes deposited from its salts before the urine leaves the body, in this case it may be passed in the form of small red crystalline masses like grains of cayenne pepper, or these may collect in the kidney or bladder to form uric acid gravel or calculi.

To ascertain if the urine contain uric acid, it is necessary to acidulate three or four fluid ounces of the urine with a fluid drachm of hydrochloric acid, or strong acetic acid, in a suitable glass vessel, an ordinary beaker being best, and to set it aside, covered with a glass plate, for 24 or 48 hours. At the end of that time, if uric acid be present, reddish-brown crystals will be seen attached to the sides and bottom of the glass, or floating on the surface of the fluid. These crystals have the flat rhombic, oval, or hexagonal shape of uric acid; they are soluble in alkalies, and give with nitric acid and ammonia the murexide test. (See below).

It has lately been shown that all the urates can be precipitated from urine by saturation with ammonium chloride. Under certain circumstances this method is very convenient; the urates thrown down in this way can readily be submitted to the murexide test, or they may be weighed, if it is required to estimate the quantity of uric acid present in a specimen of urine.

The Murexide Test.—A small portion of the suspected sediment is placed in a porcelain dish, and a drop of nitric acid let fall upon it; the dish is then gently warmed over a lamp until all the nitric acid be driven off, when, if uric acid be present, a beautiful red staining is seen; after cooling, a drop of caustic ammonia should be allowed to flow over the reddened spot, which then becomes purple; if liquor potassæ be used instead of ammonia, the colour will be violet. The test does not, however, distinguish uric acid from its salts.

Clinical Import.—The excretion of uric acid or of urates is usually increased *pari passu* with the urea in pyrexia, in acute rheumatism, and in chronic liver diseases, and in constipation. It is increased out of pro-

portion to the urea in leucæmia. Any cause
tending to diminish the urinary water, such
as free perspiration, will cause a separation
of urates from the urine on cooling, and so
produce an apparent increase in their amount.
An excess of uric acid is observed after an
attack of gout; it is often entirely absent
from the urine immediately before the paroxysm, and may disappear for days when
this disease has become chronic.

The presence of free uric acid is no proof
that uric acid is being excreted in excess;
the only inference that can be made, is that
the urine is extremely acid. But if free uric
acid shew itself immediately after the urine
has been passed, it is not improbable that a
deposit may be taking place in the pelvis of
the kidney, or the bladder—a state of considerable danger, since it may lay the found-
ation of a calculus; uric acid calculi being
the most common of all urinary concretions.

HIPPURIC ACID.

The method of preparing hippuric acid
from human urine is troublesome, and will

rarely be required to be used by the clinical student.

Take 250 c.c. or ten fluid ounces of urine, evaporate on a water bath to one-fifth of its bulk, acidify strongly with acetic acid, then stir in enough plaster of paris to make the mixture set dry and firm. When set, powder the mass and exhaust with ether. On evaporation of the ether, the hippuric acid will be left.

Hippuric acid, when evaporated to dryness with nitric acid, in a porcelain crucible, over a lamp, and then further heated to redness, gives off a gas smelling like oil of bitter almonds. This reaction is common to benzoic and hippuric acids. The crystals of hippuric acid, seen under a microscope, are long and needle-shaped prisms.

Clinical Import.—Hippuric acid exists in small quantity in the urine in health; its amount is greatly increased by the eating of much fruit, especially cranberries and greengages, and also by the ingestion of benzoic acid. The hippuric acid appears in the urine in quantity equivalent to the benzoic acid taken. Excluding these circumstances, hippuric acid is also found in quantity in the urine of fever patients, and may even be the cause of the acid reaction ; but it exists for the most part in the form of hippurates of potash and soda.

The amount is also increased in diabetes and chorea.

Nothing is known of the importance of this acid for therapeutics or diagnosis. In health the amount varies from 7 to 15 grains in the twenty-four hours.

CHLORIDES.

Chlorides may be shown to be present by the following test. To a fluid drachm of urine in a test tube, a drop of nitric acid is added, and then a few drops of a solution of nitrate of silver ; if a trace of chloride be present, a cloudiness only will be given ; but if any quantity, a white precipitate is thrown down, soluble in caustic ammonia, and re-precipitated thence by the addition of nitric acid in excess.

The nitric acid is added at first to prevent the precipitation of the phosphates with the chlorides.

A rough comparative idea of the quantity of chloride present may be made from day to day, by always taking the same quantity of urine, acidulating it in a test tube with nitric acid, and adding a solution of nitrate of silver until no further precipitate be formed. The test tube must then be set aside for twenty-four hours, and a note then taken of the proportion of the chloride of silver deposit, for comparison with other observations.

On an average, a healthy man secretes 250 grains of chloride of sodium in the twenty-four hours.

Clinical Import.—During acute pneumonia, acute rheumatism, and most other pyrexial diseases, the chlorides diminish in quantity, or even disappear from the urine. Their reappearance in daily increasing quantity is a sign of the diminution of the intensity of the disease. The amount of chlorides apparently depends upon the digestive powers of the patient even in chronic diseases.

PHOSPHATES.

The phosphates of the urine consist chiefly of acid sodium phosphate NaH_2PO_4 and acid calcium phosphate $Ca2H_2PO_4$. The corresponding salts of potassium and of magnesium are also present, though in smaller quantities. All these bodies are readily soluble in acid urine. When the urine is alkaline the phosphates of lime and magnesia are no longer in the form of the acid salts, and being insoluble are precipitated, usually in an amorphous state, though the calcium phosphate may occur in crystals as well.

If the alkalinity of the urine be due to ammonia, a crystalline compound of ammonio-magnesian phosphate is formed,

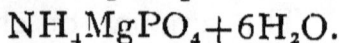

$$NH_4MgPO_4 + 6H_2O.$$

The precipitate of phosphates which is produced when a neutral urine is boiled (p. 19) is phosphate of lime; and it is probably due to a temporary conversion of the acid calcium phosphate into the insoluble neutral salt. When the urine is set aside to cool, the precipitate may redissolve, by a reconversion to its original state.

The presence of phosphates in the urine may be ascertained by the following test. A fluid is prepared by adding a drop or two of caustic ammonia to a fluid drachm of a solution of sulphate of magnesia in a test tube; hydrochloric acid is added until the precipitate caused by the ammonia be re-dissolved. Caustic ammonia is again added in excess until the fluid be strongly am-moniacal. A fluid ounce of urine is now poured into another test tube, and rendered ammoniacal with caustic ammonia; to this urine some of the prepared solution is added, and a crystalline precipitate of the ammonio-magnesian phosphate occurs at once, if the urine contain the ordinary amount of phos-phates; but the precipitate forms slowly, if the phosphates are present in very small amount.

The quantity of phosphoric acid excreted by a healthy man in the twenty-four hours is about 50 grains.

Clinical Import.—The amount of phosphoric acid in the urine is increased in diseases of the nervous centres, and of the bones, and

F

after great mental application. Acute febrile diseases cause increase of the phosphoric acid from increased tissue-metamorphosis, while in Bright's disease and some other forms of dyspepsia, the quantity of the phosphates is diminished. Dr. Gee and Dr. Zuelzer have pointed out that the phosphates diminish or disappear after the acme of the paroxysm in ague, and after some other febrile disorders.

SULPHATES.

The sulphates are at once recognised by the addition to some of the urine, in a test-tube, of a drop of hydrochloric acid, and afterwards of a few drops of a solution of chloride of barium ; a white precipitate, insoluble in nitric acid, is thrown down.

The quantity of sulphuric acid excreted by a healthy man in the twenty-four hours is about 30 grains.

Clinical Import.—The quantity of the sulphates is increased by a full animal diet or by the ingestion of any foods which contain sulphur.   Very little is known for certain of their amount in disease, and that little is at present of not much importance.

URINARY SEDIMENTS.

When a urinary deposit is to be examined, about four or five fluid ounces of the urine should be collected in a tall glass, and set aside for a few hours. If conical vessels are used, some of the sediment may cling to the sides, and this is an objection; but on the other hand their shape is advantageous because the sediment which does fall to the bottom is concentrated into a very small compass. Conical glasses are therefore preferred by some, and cylindrical glasses are more in favour with others.

If crystals form and adhere to the sides of the glass, they may very conveniently be dislodged by a glass rod with half an inch of soft rubber tubing stretched over the end, with this they can be rubbed off under the surface of the fluid, and collected at the bottom.

The sediment is to be taken up in a glass pipette, and this operation is easier if the bulk of the supernatant fluid be first poured off. A drop of the fluid containing the sediment is then to be placed on a glass slide, and covered with a cover glass. All superfluous moisture around the edge of the cover glass must be removed with a piece of blotting paper.

The sediment must be examined with a low power of the microscope first, and afterwards with a high power.

Sediments may conveniently be divided into two groups, organised and unorganised. To the latter belong uric acid, urates, oxalate of lime, phosphates, cystin, &c. ; to the former, pus, blood, mucus and epithelium, renal casts, fungi and spermatozoa.

UNORGANISED SEDIMENTS.

URIC ACID.

Uric acid is only met with as a deposit in very acid urine, and is often accompanied

by a considerable sediment of urates. Owing
to its peculiar colour and appearance, like
cayenne pepper, it can at once be recognised
by the naked eye. It is never deposited
from the urine in colourless crystals.

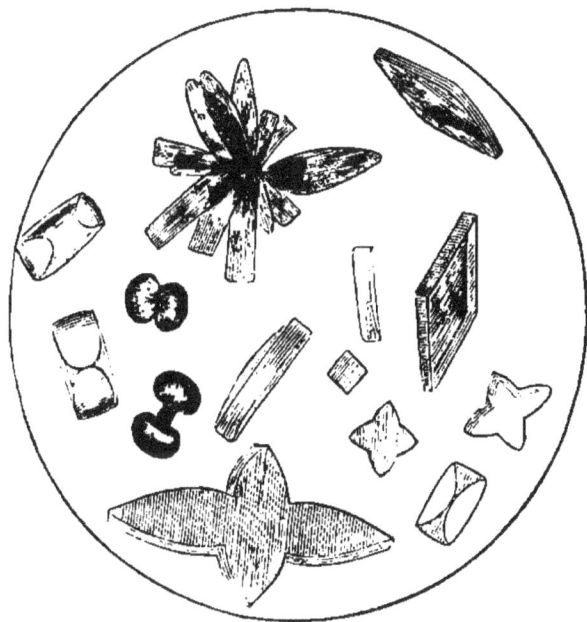

Fig. 6.—Uric Acid.

When the sediment is examined under the
microscope, the crystals are at once known
to be uric acid by their reddish-brown colour,
all other crystalline deposits being transparent and colourless. If, indeed, the student
be in doubt as to the nature of a crystal, he

will never be very wrong, if he judge it to be
uric acid when there is any tinge of brown
visible. The crystals, themselves, have numerous shapes. The most typical is that of
a lozenge or ace of diamonds, but there are
many varieties, the most common modifica-

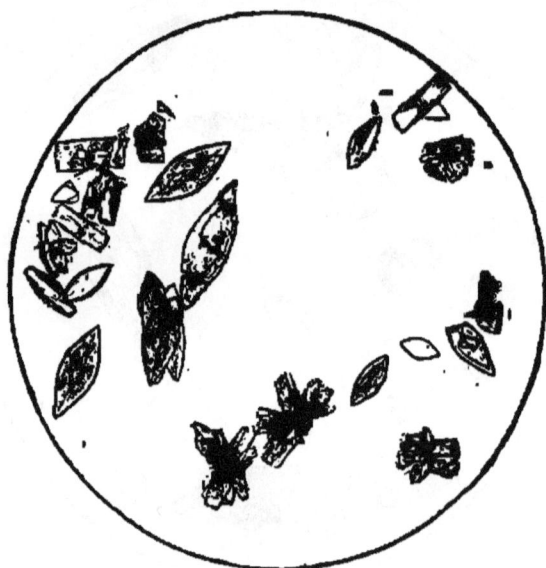

Fig. 7.—Uric Acid.

tion is for the crystals to have curved surfaces,
as a consequence of their formation in a fluid
containing uncrystallisable organic matter.
Again the lozenge shape may be a long and
slender one, or may be short and broad.
When several crystals are united together,

rosettes are formed, dumb-bells and comb-shaped masses are also sometimes found. A barrel-shaped crystal is not uncommonly met with, having two curved optical lines crossing it (see figs. 6, 7, 8).

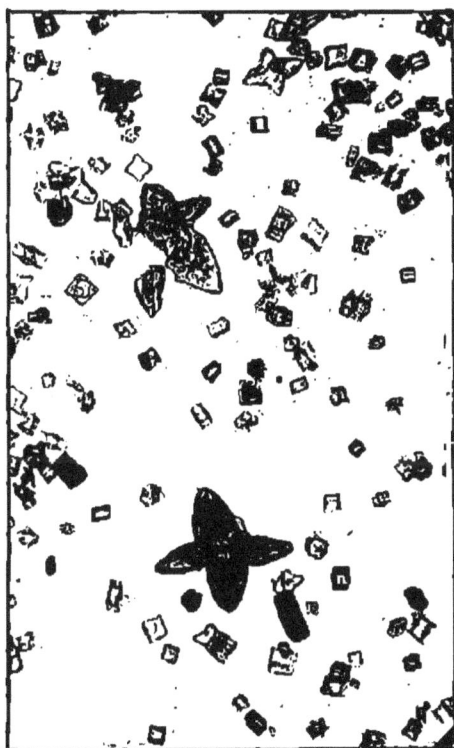

Fig. 8.—Uric Acid.

When a sediment is suspected from its appearance under the microscope to be uric acid, a chemical test can easily be applied by running in a few drops of liquor potassæ under the cover-glass. This will dissolve the crystals of uric acid, which can again be reprecipitated by adding a drop of hydrochloric or acetic acid.

The murexide test can also be applied to the sediment, see above (p. 59).

URATES.

This deposit is the most common and least important of all the urinary sediments. Any febrile state will lead to this deposit; even a greater amount of perspiration than usual will be followed by urine that becomes turbid on cooling, merely as a result of a diminished secretion of water. Urine containing an excess of urates is rarely turbid when passed; it is only when the urine is cooled, that the peculiar muddiness is observed. If the urine be gently warmed, the turbidity immediately disappears. The urates differ in colour considerably, according to the amount of colouring matter in the urine, varying from white to pink, yellow or red. In young children the "milky" urine which alarms mothers, is due to a deposit of peculiar white urates.

In the urine uric acid is found combined
with potash, with soda, with ammonia, and
with lime. The urate of soda is the most
common of the three, and is usually seen
under the microscope as an amorphous deposit; sometimes it forms small spheres with
short spikes projecting from them (fig. 9). The
urate of ammonia is rarer and occurs in
globular forms grouped together (fig. 10). It is a

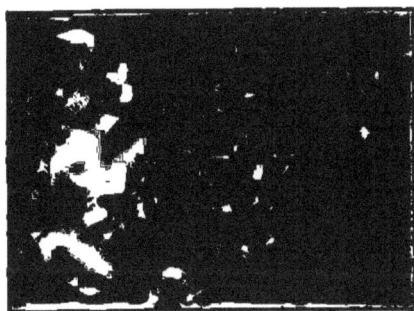

FIG. 9.—Hedgehog Crystals of Urate of Soda.

common constituent of the precipitate formed
in ammoniacal urine. The urate of lime is
very rare, and forms only an amorphous
sediment. If any doubt be entertained as to
the nature of these salts, it is necessary to
add a drop of hydrochloric or strong acetic
acid to the specimen, when crystals of uric
acid will immediately be formed. These

crystals are again dissolved by caustic soda or potash. If further evidence be required, the murexide test with nitric acid and ammonia (page 59) may be applied to them.

Sir William Roberts has shown that the urates which occur as a sediment in the urine are acid urates and contain a large percentage of very loosely combined uric

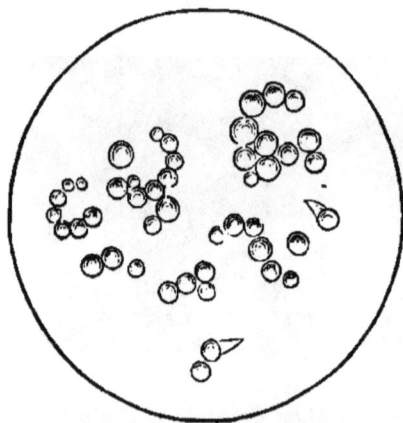

FIG. 10.—Urate of Ammonia.

acid. The combination can be readily split up, by the addition of distilled water to the sediment after it has been partly freed from urine by means of blotting paper. To carry out the experiment, let some of the sediment fall from a pipette on to thick white blotting paper. When the moisture has been absorbed, transfer the residue to a glass slide, cover it with a cover-slip, and examine it with a microscope, then run in a drop or two of distilled water, and the formation of crystals of uric acid from the amorphous urates can be observed ; this reaction may be used as a simple test for urates.

OXALATE OF LIME.

Oxalate of lime occurs as a urinary sediment in the form of minute colourless octahedral crystals. It is usually associated with the presence of an increased amount of mucus in the urine; its presence is often indicated by the unusually dense white appearance of the cloud of mucus which commonly settles from urine after standing, therefore, when the mucus forms a white conspicuous cloud in the urine glass the presence of oxalate of lime should be suspected.

The shape of the crystals is a very definite one, they consist of two four-sided pyramids springing from one base. In certain positions of the crystals the contours of the two

pyramids seem almost to coincide, producing an appearance which has been compared
to that of a square envelope, with its dia-
gonal folds (fig. 11).

Sometimes colourless dumb-bell-shaped
crystals are found associated with the octahe-
dra of oxalate of lime. These are commonly
considered to be oxalate of lime too, but

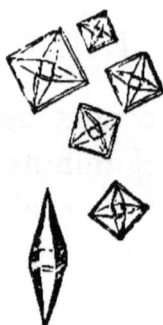

FIG. 11.—Oxalate of Lime.

they may be crystals of an allied salt, the
oxalurate of lime (fig. 12).

Oxalate of lime is insoluble in acetic acid ;
by this it is distinguished from the phosphates;
it is colourless and insoluble in alkalies, and
thus differs from uric acid. It is, however,
soluble in the mineral acids, as, for example,
in hydrochloric acid.

Clinical Import.—After urates, oxalate of

lime is the most common unorganised urinary sediment; it is often seen in the urine of patients convalescent from acute diseases; and many writers state that it may always be found when there is lessened oxidation, as in bronchitis. The occasional presence of a few crystals of oxalate of lime is not of

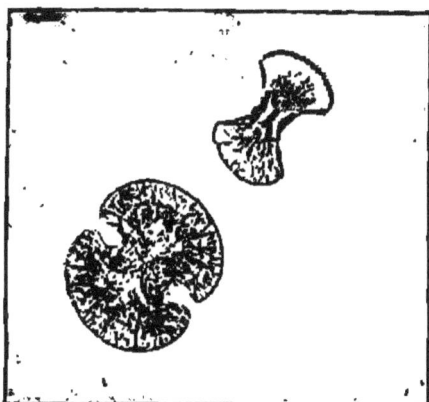

FIG. 12.—Dumb-bells of Oxalate of Lime. (From a photograph, highly magnified).

much importance. They are frequently seen in the urine after the eating of fresh fruit and vegetables. The ingestion of foods or drugs containing either oxalic acid or lime salts may cause them to appear in the urine. When the deposit is constant, and in large quantity, the formation of the mulberry calculus may be feared. This sediment is said to be associated with a dyspeptic and hypochondriacal condition, sometimes termed the "oxalic acid diathesis."

PHOSPHATES.

The phosphates are only separated from alkaline, or very feebly acid, urine; and they are always deposited when the urine undergoes the alkaline fermentation. They consist of the ammoniaco-magnesian phosphate, and the phosphate of lime. Both are usually found together.

Under the microscope, the ammoniaco-magnesian phosphate appears in beautiful right rhombic prisms, which disappear immediately on the addition of acetic acid, and are thus distinguished from the oxalate of lime with which an inexperienced observer might, perhaps, confound them.

When the ammonio-magnesian phosphate is precipitated artificially from urine by the addition of the "magnesia mixture" (p. 65) the crystals are usually branched and feathery; these "feathery phosphates"

may rarely occur in urine which has become ammoniacal through fermentation of
its urea.

Phosphate of lime usually occurs as an
amorphous precipitate, but occasionally crystals of hydrated phosphate of urine may be
seen, they form stellate groups of colourless
prisms; and are known as "stellar phosphates."

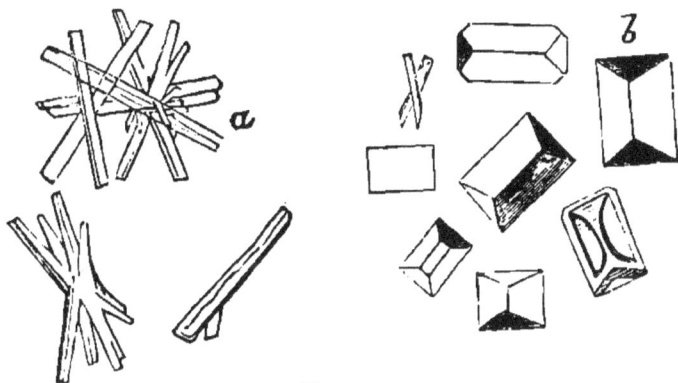

FIG. 13.

(*a*) Stellar phosphates.   (*b*) Triple phosphates.

Clinical Import.—The deposit of phosphates
indicates an alkaline reaction of the urine, a
condition favourable to the formation of
phosphatic calculi.

If the least doubt be left upon the observer's
mind after the examination of a sediment
with the microscope, he must use the aid of

reagents in determining its nature. The
following scheme will be found useful; a
drop of strong acetic acid should be placed
on the glass slide, near the thin covering
glass, so that the acid may run in between
the two pieces of glass, but it should be carefully prevented from wetting the under surface of the cover, as this will produce an
obscurity over the object. Or after having
placed a drop of the fluid containing the
sediment upon the glass slide, the end of a
thread should be placed in the drop, and
then the covering glass laid upon it, so that
the other end remains free; the acid or other
reagent may then be placed upon the free
end of the thread, and is thus conducted
along the thread to the sediment under the
cover. Should the deposit be phosphatic,
the acid quickly dissolves the crystals, or
amorphous sediment; but if the sediment
consist of urates, crystals possessing the
well-known shape of uric acid are formed.
If no effect upon the sediment is produced by
acetic acid, it consists of either uric acid or
oxalate of lime. Liquor potassæ, added with
the same precautions as acetic acid, brings
about a solution of the crystals of uric acid,

but the alkali has no effect upon the oxalate of lime, which will be dissolved by the action of hydrochloric acid.

These tests can also be applied to fragments of calculi.

CYSTIN.

Cystin is a rare deposit in the urine; it occurs in regular colourless hexagonal plates,

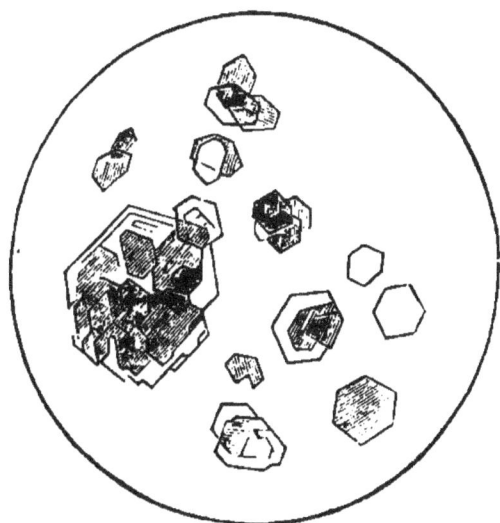

FIG. 14.—Cystin.

united by their flat surfaces, and overlapping one another. When dissolved in the urine,

G

cystin may be thrown down by the addition of acetic acid, and the precipitate examined under the microscope. It may be distinguished from uric acid, which sometimes crystallizes in hexagonal plates, by the absence of colour in the crystals.

Cystin is soluble in strong ammonia. If certain urinary crystals are suspected to be cystin the sediment containing them may be treated with a ten per cent. solution of liquor ammoniæ and the mixture filtered and set aside in a watch glass. When the ammonia has evaporated the six-sided crystals of cystin will be left behind, if cystin were present. A trace of sodium nitro-prusside gives a violet colour if added to an alkaline solution of cystin.

Cystin contains a large quantity of sulphur, and Liebig proposed a test which is founded on this fact. A solution is made by adding liquor potassæ or liquor sodæ to a small quantity of solution of acetate of lead until the precipitate first formed be redissolved; about equal parts of this solution and of urine are boiled, when black sulphide of lead is formed from the combination of the sulphur with the lead. This test is, however, by no means a good one, since many bodies frequently present in the urine, for example albumen, contain enough sulphur to give the reaction.

Clinical import.—Nothing certain is known. Sometimes cystin is found in several members of a family; and persons apparently healthy may excrete cystin for years. There is always a risk that such cases may develop cystin calculi.

LEUCIN AND TYROSIN.

Leucin and Tyrosin are very rare deposits in the urine. Under the microscope, leucin appears in dark globular crystals, which have been compared to oil drops; tyrosin, however, crystallizes in beautiful bundles of delicate needles, sometimes arranged in a sheaf-like or stellate form.

These bodies have been occasionally detected in the urine as a sediment, in cases of acute yellow atrophy of the liver.

If these bodies do not occur as a sediment, they may be looked for by the following method: a large quantity of the urine must have a solution of acetate of lead added to it so long as a precipitate forms. Through the filtrate, sulphuretted hydrogen is passed to remove the excess of lead; and the fluid is filtered again, evaporated over a water bath to a syrup, and set aside to cool; crystals of

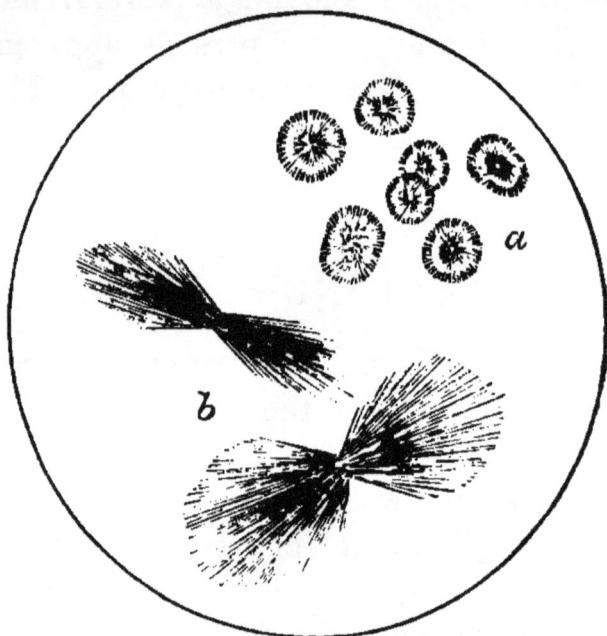

FIG 15.—(*a*) Leucin. (*b*) Tyrosin.

leucin and tyrosin will form in the viscid mass, and can be recognised under the microscope. To separate them, the residue must be treated with hot alcohol, this dissolves the leucin, leaving the tyrosin behind.

The part insoluble in spirit may now be

dissolved in water and boiled with a few drops of mercuric nitrate solution ; if tyrosin be present, the fluid becomes rose red and soon after a red precipitate is thrown down. This test for tyrosin is called Hoffmann's test, and is said to be very delicate.

The solution in spirit contains the impure leucin and requires further preparation. It must again be filtered, evaporated to dryness, and dissolved in ammonia, and then acetate of lead added so long as a precipitate forms, then filtered and washed with a little water. The precipitate on the filter, which is a combination of leucin with lead, is suspended in water, and sulphuretted hydrogen passed through, the liquid again filtered, evaporated, and set aside to crystallize. The crystals that form must be tested in the following manner : They are carefully heated with nitric acid in a platinum crucible : if leucin be present, a colourless, almost invisible, residue is left, which, warmed with a few drops of soda solution, becomes of a yellow colour passing into brown. Another test is this; if leucin be heated in a dry test tube, oily drops are formed which give off the smell of amylamin.

This preparation is undoubtedly long and troublesome; but without it, it is impossible to speak with confidence of the presence of leucin and tyrosin; of course, if a sediment suspected to be leucin or tyrosin be found in the urine, it may be tested at once by the reactions given above. But the recognition of crystals under the microscope, having the same form as leucin and tyrosin, is of small value, as in many cases, whether in health or disease, the urine may give crystals identical in form with leucin and tyrosin, but in which chemical tests altogether fail, or give the well-known reactions of other bodies.

Clinical import.—Leucin and tyrosin occur in the urine of acute yellow atrophy of the liver, and of phosphorus poisoning. They have been said to occur in acute tuberculosis, in typhus fever and in small-pox.

ORGANISED SEDIMENTS.

BLOOD.

If blood be present in the urine in abundance, there may be a brown or reddish sediment of blood corpuscles mixed with fibrin to form a clot. In such a case the sediment will give the reactions and tests for blood which have been already described, and a microscopic examination of the sediment will show abundance of red-blood corpuscles. The Hæmin test may also be applied as follows. Transfer a small portion of the sediment to a slide, and dry it by gentle heat, add a crystal or two of chloride of sodium, and two drops of glacial acetic acid, cover with a cover glass and heat to ebullition over a small spirit lamp flame; when cold, examine under the microscope for the small reddish-brown rhomboidal crystals of hæmin.

Another method of detecting blood in a sediment is to treat it with alcohol to which a few minims of liquor ammoniæ have been added; it should be boiled for two or three minutes and filtered; to the filtrate add a few drops of ammonium sulphide, and examine with a spectroscope for the two bands of reduced hæmatin.

These tests are seldom needed for the detection of blood in urine, for if there be enough blood present to produce a sediment the ordinary tests for blood will readily prove its presence in the supernatant fluid.

PUS.

Pus is often present in the urine, and forms a thick sediment at the bottom of the urine glass. The urine readily becomes alkaline, and rapidly decomposes after being passed. It is permanently turbid; that is, the turbidity is unaffected by heat.

Under the microscope, the deposit shows numerous pus corpuscles, round colourless bodies, not varying much in size, having granular contents, and nuclei varying from one to four in number; if acted on by acetic acid, the nuclei become much more distinct. If the urine have been long passed, the pus corpuscles undergo changes which render them incapable of being recognised.

The urine of course contains albumen, and in proportion to the amount of pus present. If the quantity of albumen exceed that which should be given by the pus present in the

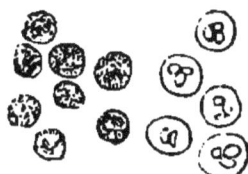

Fig. 16.—Pus corpuscles in urine, unaltered, and affected by acetic acid.

urine, evidence of kidney disease, as casts of tubes, should at once be looked for.

The deposit from urine containing pus is rendered viscid and gelatinous by the addition of about half its quantity of liquor potassæ; it becomes ropy and falls in a mass when dropped from one vessel to the other; urine containing mucus on the other hand, becomes more fluid and limpid by the addition of caustic alkali.

Pus occurs in the urine in the following diseases :—

Leucorrhœa in women.

Gonorrhœa or Gleet in men.

Pyelitis, from any cause.

Cystitis.

Any abscess bursting into any part of the urinary tract.

Leucorrhœa is an exceedingly frequent cause of the presence of a slight amount of albumen in the urine of women ; if it be necessary to exclude this origin, the urine must be obtained by means of the catheter.

MUCUS AND EPITHELIUM.

Mucus is a constant constituent of every urine, and if healthy urine be allowed to remain at rest for an hour, a light cloud will be found floating in the fluid or settled at the bottom of the urine glass; on examination with the microscope, it will be found to consist of amorphous particles mixed with corpuscles and epithelium scales detached from the surfaces over which the urine has passed. The mucus is increased in quantity

in catarrhal conditions of the urinary tract.
It is dissolved by dilute alkalies and precipitated from its solutions by acetic or other
dilute acids; on this account it forms a
cloud in acid urines; in alkaline urines it
may be present in solution, and if abundant,
it may be thrown down on acidification, and
so simulate albumen.

Dr. George Oliver has examined the reactions of mucin in the urine, and finds that
both potassio-mercuric iodide and picric acid
will give a turbidity with mucin. In acid
urines the mucin is in suspension, and can
be removed by filtration before the tests for
albumen are applied, but in alkaline urines
the mucin is in solution, and cannot be got
rid of in this way. Moreover the urines
which contain an excess of mucin are often
alkaline in reaction. In these cases it is
best to acidify the urine very slightly with
dilute acetic acid to precipitate the mucin,
which can then be separated by filtration.

Dr. Oliver recommends the following test
with his prepared papers : to a drachm of
urine add a citric acid paper and a potassio-
mercuric iodide paper. A slight milkiness

which disappears on warming and returns on cooling signifies the presence of mucin.

The urethra and bladder give up a round-ish or oval epithelium cell to the urine. In the urine of women, especially in cases of

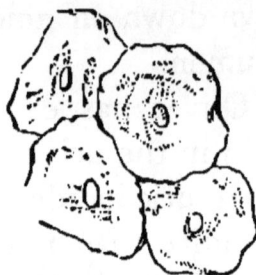

Fig. 17.—Vaginal epithelium.

leucorrhœa, the epithelium cells of the vagina are very numerous; they exactly resemble the squamous epithelium of the mouth. Under irritation, the mucous membrane of the renal pelvis and ureter will produce cells, caudate, spindle-shaped, and irregular, very like those formerly looked upon as diagnostic of cancer. From this circumstance it is impossible to speak positively of the existence of cancer cells in the urine.

Desquamation of the tubular epithelium of the kidney occurs only in disease; the cells, as seen in the urine, are slightly swollen,

and acquire a more spheroidal, and less
distinctly polygonal shape, apparently from
the imbibition of fluid, and the removal of
pressure. The cells are frequently gran-

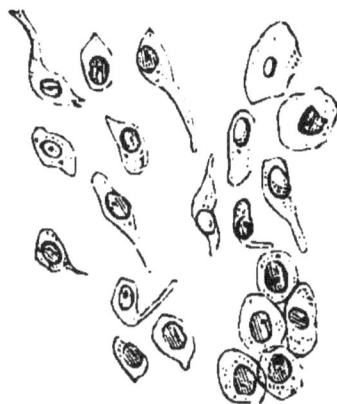

FIG. 18.—Epithelium from the bladder, ureter and pelvis of
the kidney.

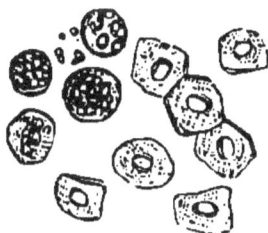

FIG. 19.—Renal epithelium, healthy and fatty.

ular and contain fat drops, or are contracted,
withered up, and shrivelled.

Clinical import.—See Section on Renal
Casts below.

RENAL CASTS.

In Bright's disease and in congestion of the kidney, there are formed in the uriniferous tubules lengthened cylinders which are discharged with the urine, and form the deposit known as "casts." Those found in the urine are probably chiefly formed in the straight uriniferous tubes; and there are two views of the origin of renal casts: one is that casts are formed by the escape of blood or plasma into the tubes of the kidney, and coagulation of the fibrin, which thus becomes moulded to the shape of the tube into which it has been extravasated. It is possible that many of the hyaline casts are formed in this way. The other view is that the epithelial and granular casts are produced by a desquamation and degeneration of the renal epithelium.

When the urine contains casts in great quantity, they can scarcely be overlooked, if the urine be allowed to settle for a few hours in a tall cylindrical glass, the whole of the supernatant fluid poured off, and the last drops which flow from the lip of the glass

put under the microscope and examined. If
there be but few casts present, the whole of
the urine of the twenty-four hours should be
collected in a tall glass and allowed to settle
for about twelve ours. The urine must then
be all poured away, save the four or five
ounces which have collected at the bottom.
This residue must then be allowed to settle
again for a few hours, when if casts be present, they will be ound at the bottom of the
glass, the last drops poured away being put
under the microscope. Casts may oftentimes
be missed if the urine given for examination
be only the upper layer of a specimen which
has settled for some hours and of which all
the casts have fallen to the bottom. It thus
sometimes becomes of importance to collect
all the urine passed.

The detection of casts is very much facili-
tated by staining them. This may be readily
carried out by adding a few drops of solution
of fuchsine, or of methylene blue to the urine,
and allowing it to stand for a few hours until
the casts settle to the bottom, or a drop of
the same dyes may be added to the drop of
urine on the slide just before it is to be
examined ; the dye must be very dilute, so

as not to give more than a faint tinge of colour to the urine itself.

With a little experience, the student will soon become familiar with the appearance of casts, and will at once be able to distinguish them from foreign bodies in the urine. They are never broader than six, or less than two, red blood corpuscles in diameter ; but they vary considerably in length, never, however, exceeding the $\frac{1}{50}$ of an inch. The same cast does not vary greatly in its diameter, and never becomes twisted on itself, as a cotton fibre does.

The foreign bodies, most likely to be mistaken for renal casts, are cotton fibres, hair, and pieces of deal.

Cotton fibres have a very irregular outline and are much broader at one point than another ; they are often twisted, and of great length, which will distinguish them from casts. Their structure is often striped in a longitudinal direction.

Hair can often be distinguished from renal casts by its colour alone ; and if this be not very apparent, by its possessing a cortical and medullary structure ; and by its length being greater than that of any cast.

Fibres of deal, which have their source in furniture, flooring, &c., may perhaps be mistaken for renal casts. They are at once recognised by the presence of the large round wood cells which characterise the tribe of Coniferæ.

In the urine of female patients in the wards of a hospital a curious sedimentary deposit of round or oval bodies may sometimes prove perplexing. These bodies are starch grains derived from some form of starch powder or dusting powder applied for toilet purposes to the patients by the nurses.

Casts may be conveniently divided, according to their appearance under the microscope, into three kinds, the epithelial cast, the granular cast, and the hyaline cast.

The epithelial cast. The cylinder consists of a mass of epithelium cells derived from the tubules of the kidney ; the cells may become granular and acquire a dark appearance by transmitted light. The cast is usually wide, never very narrow.

The granular cast. This is a solid cylinder having a granular appearance, which may be limited to a few dark points in the substance of the casts, or be so intense as to give the casts an almost black appearance. In this kind of cast may often be found epithelial cells, blood corpuscles, red or white, pus corpuscles, crystals of uric acid, urates, and especially oxalate of lime. The fatty cast is a variety of the granular, produced by the running together, into globules, of the granules of fat.

The hyaline cast. This cast is usually very transparent, and the outline is often so indistinct that a little iodine or magenta must be added to the urine before it can be detected, or a diaphragm with a narrow opening must be used. They show indistinct markings on their surface, or a few granules and nuclei. There are two kinds, the wide and the narrow; the latter are sometimes of great length.

In observing casts, notice must be taken of the action of acids upon them, or their contents. The granules on the cast, if albuminous, will disappear when acted on by acetic acid; but if fatty, they are rendered more distinct. The width of the cylinder is of some importance, as it is supposed that very broad casts are formed in tubules completely stripped of their epithelium, and

that the prognosis is more grave when these
wide casts show on their sides no nuclei,
or attempt at re-formation of epithelium.
From later observations on the varying

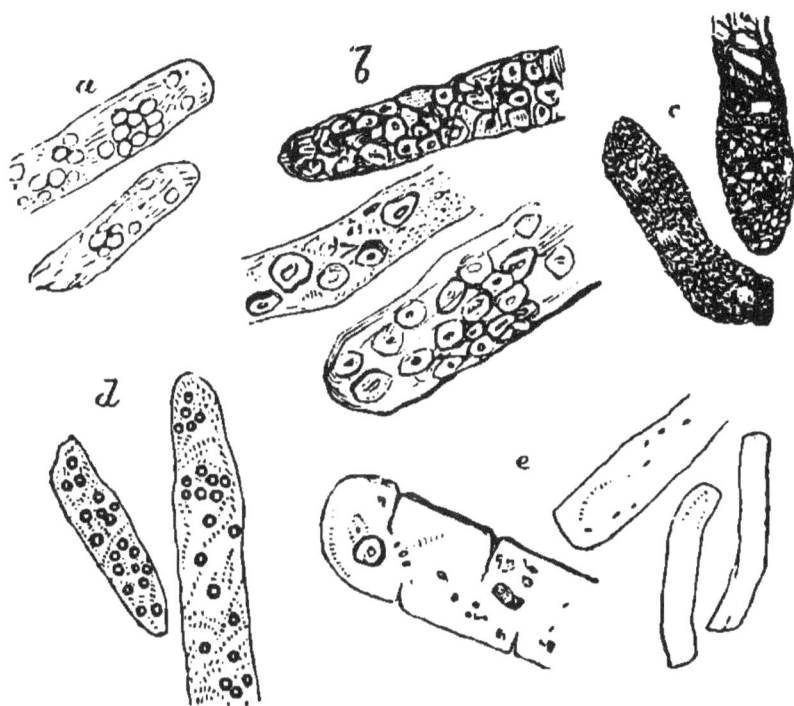

FIG. 20.—*a.* Blood casts. *b.* Epithelial casts. *c.* Granular
casts. *d.* Fatty casts. *e.* Hyaline casts.

diameters of the uriniferous tubes, the importance of the breadth of the cast becomes
less.

Occasionally casts may be seen which are

H 2

composed of masses of micrococci. They are of serious import, and generally signify that some infective process is taking place in the renal tubules.

Clinical import. The presence of casts in the urine is a sure sign of disease of the kidney, but not, however, necessarily of permanent disease of the kidney. They are present in many acute diseases, accompanied by albumen in the urine; but if they are found for several weeks together after all fever have left the patient, then permanent disease of the kidney may be inferred. Casts are constantly present in the urine in all cases of congestion of the kidney, and of acute or chronic Bright's disease. But no certain information as to the nature of the disease existing in the kidney, for example, whether lardaceous or otherwise, can be had from the characters of the casts, since all forms of Bright's disease end in fatty changes. Some help may, however, be derived from the appearance of the casts in forming a judgment of the acute or chronic character, or a prognosis, of the disease. If, for example, there be found in the urine epithelial casts which have undergone little, or no, granular change, and casts studded with red blood corpuscles, together with a large quantity of epithelium from the tubules of the kidney, having a natural or only slightly clouded appearance, there can be little doubt that the patient is suffering from an acute attack of Bright's disease ; while if the casts be chiefly fatty, or intensely granular, and the epithelium be small in amount, and the cells withered and contracted, or containing globules of oil, it will be more than probable that the case is one of chronic Bright's dis-ease.

Since little trust can be put in the characters of the casts as an aid to special diagnosis, some of the leading characters of the renal derivatives in the chief forms of kidney affection will now be spoken of more at length.

Congestion of the kidney.—The casts are chiefly hyaline, seldom showing any marks of fatty change. Very rarely may blood or epithelial casts be discovered.

Acute Bright's disease.—At the beginning, the urine deposits a sediment which consists of blood-corpuscles, narrow hyaline casts, and casts covered with blood corpuscles, the

" blood cast " of some authors. In the next stage, the amount of blood present is not so great, but a great desquamation of the renal tubules taking place, renal epithelium and epithelial casts are found in great numbers; the epithelium has undergone little, if any, granular change ; hyaline casts are observed together with epithelial. In the next stage, the changes in the epithelium may be almost daily observed; at first they become granular, cloudy in appearance, which change often goes on to fatty degeneration, and the epithelial cells then contain large fat drops, while the epithelial casts undergo a like change, and become distinctly granular and even fatty.

If the patient recover, the casts and epithelium slowly disappear from the urine, but if the case become chronic, the renal derivatives show the characters described in the next paragraph.

Chronic Bright's disease.—Numerous forms of casts are met with ; the hyaline, both narrow and wide forms ; the larger are often beset with granules dissolved on the addition of acetic acid ; the granular, whose surface is often covered with fatty or shrivelled up epithelium cells; fat drops may stud the cylinder. Epithelial casts are rare, except in febrile exacerbations, when the renal derivatives found in acute Bright's disease are present together with granular and fatty casts, evidence of this previous alteration of the kidney. .

Lardaceous or amyloid kidney.—The urinary deposit contains hyaline casts, which sometimes give the amyloid reaction, and which are often accompanied by pus corpuscles. Atrophied epithelial cells, becoming fatty in the latter stages of the disease, are almost invariably present.

MICRO-ORGANISMS.

Many kinds of organisms appear in the urine after it has been voided for some time, and when the ammoniacal decomposition has begun, or is about to begin. The most important are *micrococci* and *bacteria*. When found in freshly passed urine, they are often due to the introduction into the bladder of catheters imperfectly cleansed. It is probable that catheters are seldom properly cleansed (sterilised) after use.

When there is any fistulous communication between the rectum and bladder micro-organisms may occur in the urine.

In the various forms of general infection as by the specific fevers, erysipelas, tuberculosis, etc., the specific micro-organisms have been detected in the urine.

Sarcinæ have been seen a few times in the urine. They are characterised by their peculiar arrangement into square packets.

Penicillium glaucum or mould fungi, and *Torula cerevisiæ* or yeast fungi may develop in urine after it has been passed, especially in diabetic urine.

SPERMATOZOA.

These bodies are present in the urine of men first passed after an emission of semen. A few pass away in the urine, probably, without venereal excitement, especially when the person is continent. In the urine of women, they are almost positive proof of sexual intercourse.

The seminal secretion forms a glairy white deposit at the bottom of the urine glass. When examined with the microscope, (for which a high power, magnifying 400 or 500 diameters, is best, although a power of 250 will identify them), spermatozoa show the characteristic oval head or body often some-what pear-shaped, and long delicate tail, two or three times the length of the head. In the urine no movement is ever shewn by these bodies.

APPENDIX.

It has been thought desirable to add a short account of the method of estimating quantitatively the chief substances found in the urine, since the clinical clerk may often be desired to make an analysis of the urea, chlorides, phosphates, &c. No account of the method of making standard solutions will be given, as this preparation requires a greater knowledge of chemistry than is usually possessed by the clinical student. For the same reason, no details have been introduced which require the use of a balance.

The metric weights and measures only will be employed : they are :—

The litre, the unit for measures of capa-city $= 1\cdot 76$ pints.

The cubic centimeter, (C.C.) the $\frac{1}{1000}$ part of a litre.

The gramme, (grm.) the unit of weight, the weight of a cubic centimeter of dis-

tilled water, at 4°C. at normal baro-
meter pressure, $= 15\cdot43$ English grains.

The milligramme, the $\frac{1}{1000}$ part of a
gramme.

The apparatus will be :—

A measure of litre capacity, divided into
parts containing 10 C.C. at least.

Burettes, divided into quarters of a C.C.

Pipettes, which deliver 5, 10, 15, 20, 30
and 50 C.C.

Beakers, Berlin dishes, stirring rods, &c.

GENERAL DIRECTIONS.

The whole of the urine passed in the 24
hours must be obtained : it will be found
most convenient to collect it from 9 a.m. on
one day to 9 a.m. on the following day,
making the patient micturate just before
this hour.

The urine must be kept, as it is passed, in
a covered glass vessel. When the analysis
is to be made, the urine must be measured
in a vessel graduated to 1000 C.C. and
marked into divisions of 10 C.C. After

measuring, the whole of the urine must be mixed together, and a portion of this used in the estimation of the urea, chlorides, &c.

A complication arises if the urine contain albumen; and, in this case, the albumen must be removed before proceeding to the analysis of the urea, &c.; a measured quantity of urine, 100 or 200 C.C., is heated to the boiling point in a Berlin dish, the bottom of which is protected from the flame by a piece of iron wire gauze. If the albumen do not separate in flakes, dilute acetic acid is *very* carefully added until the acid reaction be marked. If too much acetic acid be added, part of the albumen may be redissolved. The heat must be moderate and only just rise to boiling point, or the urea will be decomposed. The urine, after cooling, is then to be filtered into the same measure that was used in the beginning to ascertain the volume (100 or 200 C.C.) the dish and filter washed with small quantities of distilled water, which are added to the filtrate, until the urine stand at exactly 100 or 200 C.C. according to the initial quantity. This fluid is then used in the estimation of the urea, chlorides, phosphates, sugar, &c.

ESTIMATION OF UREA.

There are two methods now commonly in use for the estimation of urea:—

The first process, a modification of Hüfner's, is based upon the fact that when urea is acted on by an alkaline hypobromite, nitrogen is given off, and this nitrogen, when collected and measured, gives an estimation of the quantity of urea decomposed.

The second process, first employed by Liebig, and known by his name, depends upon a reaction of urea with mercuric nitrate in which these two bodies combine to form a white precipitate. This reaction is used as the basis of a volumetric estimation of urea, which will be described below.

In both of these processes it is necessary to ascertain beforehand the presence or absence of albumen. If albumen be present it must be separated by the method given on the page above. If the urine be free from albumen, both the methods may be used without further preparation of the urine.

1. *The Hypobromite Method.*—Many forms of apparatus have been contrived for sim-

plifying the carrying out of this test; one,
introduced by Dr. Russell and Dr. Samuel
West, has been largely used for clinical work,
and will be described; a more recent, and

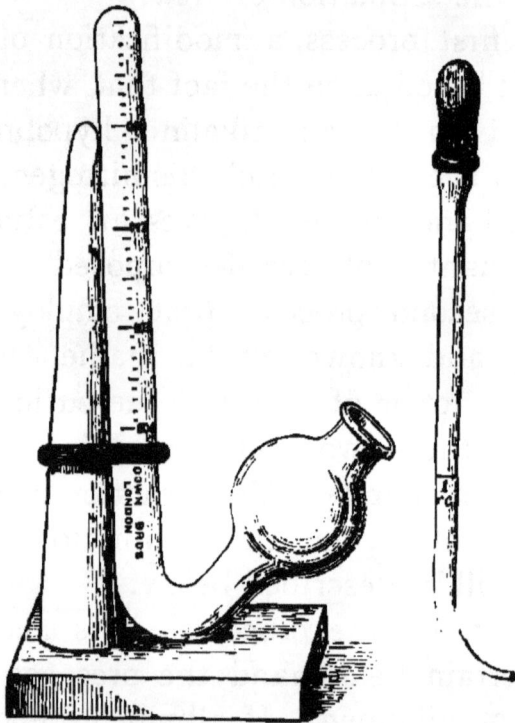

FIG. 21.—Southall's apparatus for estimation of urea.

better form of apparatus for the same pur-
pose, commonly known as Southall's apparatus, will be described first.   It consists of a
bent graduated tube closed at one end, and
expanded into a funnel at the other.   It is

supported upon a wooden stand in an inverted position, so that the gas evolved during the reaction may be collected in the graduated limb, while the liquid displaced by the gas is retained in the expanded lower portion ; the hypobromite solution is made by adding bromine to a solution of caustic soda ; it must be freshly made, as it will not keep long.

The composition of the hypobromite solution is as follows :—

Sodium hydrate, 5 parts; distilled water 20 parts ; bromine 2 fluid parts. This solution keeps well for about a month, and may be easily prepared in a moment, fresh and fresh as wanted, by keeping a quantity of sodium solution ready, and then adding the needful proportion of bromine to a measured amount of the caustic soda solution. The bromine should be kept in sealed glass capsules, which may be dropped into the solution and broken with a shake. In this way the disagreeable odour and inconvenience of handling the bromine are avoided.

The exact strength of the solution is only important in so far as this, that there must be enough hypobromite present to decompose the whole of the urea, and enough free caustic soda to absorb all the CO_2 produced by the reaction which may be written as follows:—

$$CON_2H_4 + 3NaBrO = CO_2 + N_2 + 2H_2O + 3NaBr.$$

The directions for the use of Southall's apparatus are as follows:—

Fill the vertical tube with a solution of hypobromite of sodium by pouring the solution into the bulb until it is about half full; the apparatus should then be inclined horizontally until the entire tube is filled and just a little left in the bulb (say $\frac{1}{3}$ or thereabouts); then restore the apparatus to the vertical position.

Having drawn into the pipette 1 cubic centimeter of the urine to be tested, which should be taken from the collected and measured excretion of 24 hours, the pipette is passed into the apparatus, the point being placed immediately under the long arm; the india-rubber cap is now slowly compressed, so that the urine which is liberated all passes up the long tube; as the urine passes through the solution the urea becomes decomposed and the nitrogen is set free. This gas now collects at the upper part of the tube, and its volume being measured, indicates the amount of the urea from which it is evolved. In cases where there is much urea, it is advisable to mix the urine with an equal amount of water before testing, the proportion of urea will then be equal to double of that indicated on the scale.

The graduations are arranged so as to save the necessity of calculation, and give either of two readings.

(1). *Metrical Scale.*—Each division indicates ·001 gramme of urea in 1 C.C. of urine. The percentage of urea is obtained by multiplying the result of the test by 100. To ascertain the total amount of urea voided in 24 hours, multiply the result of the test by the number of C.C. of urine passed during that period.

(2) *English Scale.*—Each division indicates one grain of urea per fluid ounce of urine. The result of the test, when multiplied by the number of ounces of urine passed in 24 hours will give the total amount of urea voided during that period.*

The apparatus† contrived by Russell and West is figured in the adjoining woodcut

---

* The apparatus may be obtained from Down Bros., 5 & 7 St. Thomas's Street, London, S.E.

† It may be had of Cetti, Brooke Street, Holborn.

(fig. 22).   It consists of the tube A, which is
about nine inches long, narrowed somewhat
before the closed end is reached, which end
is blown out into a bulb, B.   The free end is

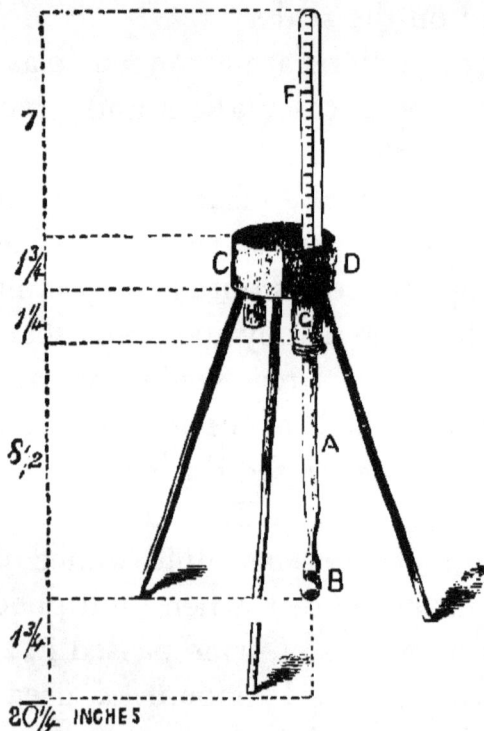

FIG. 22.

fitted by means of an india-rubber cork into
the hole G at the bottom of the trough C D
which stands on three legs.   When an estimation is to be made, 5 C.C. of urine are

measured off with a pipette and allowed to run down the side of the tube A, into the bulb B. Distilled water is then added by means of a wash-bottle, to wash away the urine adhering to the sides of the tube, but in quantity enough only to fill up the bulb as high as the constriction, or a very little above it. A glass rod tipped with india-rubber is then introduced into the tube, A, so that the india-rubber fills up the constriction and acts as a cork. Care must be taken that no air bubbles are present below the constriction. The hypobromite solution is then poured into the tube until it is quite full, and the trough is filled with common water. The graduated tube F, is then filled with water, the thumb slipped over it, so that it contains no air bubbles, and it is then inverted in the trough. The glass rod tipped with india-rubber is withdrawn, and the graduated tube, F, immediately slipped over the mouth of the tube A. The mouth of this should project well up into the tube F, so as to prevent the escape of any of the gas. The reaction begins immediately, but in order to bring it to an end as quickly as possible, the bulb should be warmed by a spirit lamp or Bun-

I 2

sen's burner, till the bulb be hot to the hand.
In five minutes the amount of gas may be
read off. After some hours the gas is lessened in quantity; it is thus important to
read it off as soon as the reaction is over.
The amount of gas measured by the divisions
on the tube gives the percentage of the urea
in the specimen of urine examined.

The estimation of the total amount of urea
excreted in the twenty-four hours is now easy.
All that is to be done is to multiply the total
number of cubic centimeters of urine passed
in the twenty-four hours by the figures read
off on the measured tube. Thus if the
amount of urine passed in twenty-four hours
be 1770 C.C. and the number of the tube
read off 1·8 it is only necessary to multiply
1770 by 18 to get the amount of urea in
milligrammes. In this case it will be 31860
milligrammes, and since 1000 milligrammes
equal one gramme, the total amount of urea
passed will be 31·86 grammes or about 1·8
per cent.

If the urine contain more than two *per cent.*
of urea, the urine must be diluted with an
equal bulk of distilled water, the test then
carried out, and the results doubled.

The hypobromite methods give fair results for clinical purposes, but they are not to be regarded as more than rough approximations. Liebig's method admits of far higher accuracy, and, as a matter of fact, it is not at all difficult to carry out, when once the burette has been set up and the standard solution provided.

The following method is that described by Liebig :—

The solutions required are :—

A standard solution of mercuric nitrate of which 1 C.C. corresponds exactly to 10 milligrammes of urea.

A solution of baryta, made by mixing two volumes of cold saturated solution of barium hydrate, with one volume of cold saturated solution of barium nitrate.

A saturated solution of carbonate of soda to be used as the indicator.

If the urine be free from albumen, a measured pipette, containing 10 or 15 C.C., is filled with urine, *twice*, and the urine allowed to run into a urine glass or beaker. The same pipette is next filled with the baryta solution which is then added to the urine previously measured off. There are thus two volumes of urine mixed with one of baryta solution. The mixture is then passed through filtering paper ; a drop or two of the filtrate is to be tested with the baryta solution to see if any further precipitate occur, and if any precipitate do occur, it is best to take a fresh quantity of urine and to add to it an *equal* volume of baryta solution ; after filtration, this must again be tested. The object of the addition of the baryta is to remove the phosphates from the urine.

The next step is to measure off a definite quantity of the filtrate, so that in any case it may contain 10 C.C. of urine. Thus, if one volume of baryta solution were used with two volumes of urine, 15 C.C. of the filtrate would be measured off with the pipette. If equal volumes of urine and baryta solution were employed, 20 C.C. must be measured off. A burette divided into quarters of a cubic centimeter is then to be filled with the standard solution of mercuric nitrate. The burette must be filled to the brim, and allowed to remain at rest for some time, so that all bubbles may rise to the surface and escape. The solution must then be let off by the pinch-cock at the bottom of the burette, until the upper surface be exactly on a level with the first division of the burette. Care must be taken that the solution fills the whole of the apparatus below the pinch-cock, and that no air bubbles are there contained : for if the latter rise to the surface during the analysis, the estimation is, of course, vitiated.

The measured quantity of the filtrate of the urine and baryta is then to be placed in a small glass vessel, a beaker holding about 100 C.C. being best ; a few drops of dilute nitric acid are to be added and the vessel placed under the burette.* The work of

---

* A great saving of time may be effected by making two separate estimations; in the first estimation, 15 C.C. of the mercury solution may at once be added to the fluid in the beaker and a drop of the mixture, after thorough stirring, is to be added to a drop of the soda solution on a white tile; if no yellow colour appear in the soda solution, continue adding the mercury solution in 5 C.C. at a time, and testing with soda after each addition, until a yellow colour is produced. The exact point for the estimation of the urea is found to be between 15 and 20 C.C. or 20 and 25 C.C., as the case may be. A second estimation is then made, and mercury solution to the amount of the smallest number of

estimating the urea now begins. The solution of nitrate of mercury is allowed to run, drop by drop, into the fluid below, stirring the latter well with a glass rod, until a permanent precipitate be produced; the absence, at first, of a permanent precipitate is caused by the chlorides present; the amount of nitrate of mercury used is then read off and noted down; the nitrate of mercury is then added by quarters or halves of a C.C. the mixture being well stirred after every addition, until a drop of the mixture give a yellow colour when brought into contact with the solution of carbonate of soda.

A convenient method of recognising the first appearance of the yellow colour is to place a glass plate on a piece of black paper, with a few drops of saturated solution of carbonate of soda spread over it; and to let fall as small a drop as possible of the fluid from the beaker into the margin of the soda solution. If no yellow colour be seen, another half C.C. of the mercury solution

---

C.C. *before* the yellow colour was produced, is at once allowed to flow into the beaker, and then added more carefully by quarters or halves of a C.C. as described in the text.

must be added, and the fluid from the beaker again tested with the soda, and the mercury solution must be added, until the least appearance of yellow occur, when one drop more of the mercury solution must be added to the beaker, the fluid well stirred about, and another small drop taken from the mixture and tested with the soda, when if the process have been rightly performed, an increase in the yellow colour will be perceived. Great care must be taken during the whole of these operations, not to lose one single drop of the fluid from either the beaker or burette. The number of C.C. used is then read off.

From the total number of C.C. used, there must be subtracted the number of C.C. used in the first part of the process before a permanent precipitate was produced, and the remainder multiplied by 10 gives the number of milligrammes of urea contained in 10 C.C. of urine, because 1 C.C. of the mercury solution corresponds to 10 milligrammes of urea.

Thus far the amount of urea contained in 10 C.C. of urine has been ascertained; by simple proportion it is easy to find the quantity passed in the twenty-four hours. For example, suppose that 1 C.C. of the mercury solution were used before a permanent precipitate was produced; and that 19 C.C. were used before the yellow colour was distinctly seen, then 1 C.C. subtracted from 19 C.C. leaves 18, which multiplied by 10 gives 180 milligrammes of urea in 10 C.C. of urine. Suppose that the patient had passed 1770 C.C. of urine in the twenty-four hours, then the calculation would be as follows:—

$$10 : 1770 : : 180 : 31860$$
$$180$$

$$10) \overline{318600}$$

$$31860 \text{ milligrammes.}$$

As 1000 milligrammes equal 1 gramme, 31860 milligrammes equal 31·860 grammes. To obtain the percentage of urea proceed as follows:—

1 per cent. in 1770 C.C. is 17·7 grm.

$$17·7 : 31·86 \text{ as } 1 : x$$

x being the percentage required.

ESTIMATION OF CHLORIDES.

The solutions required are :—

A standard solution of nitrate of silver, of which 1 C.C. corresponds exactly to 10 milligrammes of chloride of sodium.

A saturated solution of neutral chromate of potash.

The urine should be as fresh as possible, and, if albuminous, submitted to the preparation described at page 108. 10 C.C. of urine are then measured off into a glass vessel or beaker, and two or three drops of the solution of chromate of potash added. A burette divided into quarters of a C.C. is then filled with the standard solution of nitrate of silver, and the precautions as to filling burettes, described in speaking of the estimation of urea (p. 118) must be observed. The silver solution must then be allowed to fall into the beaker, and each drop well mixed with the urine by means of a glass rod. As each drop falls into the urine, it must be carefully watched for the least tinge of red surrounding the precipitate of chloride of silver. This reddish colour announces the approaching termination of the process, and is at first not permanent, but disappears when the fluid in the beaker is well stirred. The first drop, however, which produces a reddish tinge not disappearing by agitation, indicates that the whole of the chloride present has been precipitated, and that chromate of silver is beginning to be formed. The quantity of silver solution used is now read off, and another drop let fall into the beaker from the burette, when the reddish colour ought to be heightened. From the number of C.C. used, the quantity of chloride is calculated ; for, since 1 C.C. of the silver solution corresponds to 10 milligrammes of chloride of sodium, the number of C.C. of the silver solution used, multiplied by 10, will give the amount in milligrammes of the chloride of sodium present in 10 C.C. of urine. Thus if 6 C.C. of silver solution were used before a permanent reddish precipitate was produced, 10 C.C. of urine will contain 60 milligrammes of chloride of sodium, and if the patient passed 1200 C.C. of urine in the twenty-four hours, the amount of chloride passed can be easily calculated in the following way :—

$$10 : 1200 : : 60 : 7200$$

7200 milligrammes equal 7·2 grammes which will be the total quantity passed in the twenty-four hours.

This process, as applied to urine, nearly always gives a result a little above the real amount present.

For greater accuracy, therefore 10 C.C. of the urine are measured off into a porcelain crucible, 1 or 2 grammes of nitrate of potash free from chlorides, are dissolved in it, and the whole slowly evaporated to dryness, and exposed to a low red heat, until the carbon be completely oxydised, and the contents of the crucible white. After cooling, these are dissolved in distilled water, a few drops of nitric acid added until a faintly acid reaction be produced, a small quantity of carbonate of lime being then added in order to make the solution again neutral, the solution filtered, and the chlorides then estimated in the manner described above.

The reaction referred to in the estimation of urea by mercuric nitrate, namely, that chlorides prevent the white precipitate of mercuric nitrate with urea, can also be used as a method of estimating the chlorides in urine. See Harris and Power, *Handbook for the Physiological Laboratory*, 5th edit., 1892.

ESTIMATION OF PHOSPHATES.

The solutions required are :—

A standard solution of acetate of uranium, of which 1 C.C. corresponds exactly to 5 milligrammes of phosphoric acid.

A solution containing acetic acid and acetate of soda : 100 grammes of acetate of soda are dissolved in water, 100 C.C. of acetic acid added, and the mixture diluted until it equal 1000 C.C.

A weak solution of ferrocyanide of potassium.

50 C.C. of the filtered urine are mixed in a beaker with 5 C.C. of the solution of acetic acid and acetate of soda. The beaker is placed over a water bath, and when the mixture is well warmed, the standard uranium solution is dropped into the beaker until

precipitation cease ; this can easily be ascertained by allowing the solution to trickle down the side of the beaker. A small drop from the beaker is then to be placed on a porcelain dish by means of a glass rod, and a drop of the solution of ferrocyanide of potassium placed close to it by means of another glass rod and the two drops allowed to run together. If no alteration of the colour be produced at their line of meeting, more of the uranium solution must be added to the urine, until a drop tested with the solution of ferrocyanide of potassium, produce a light brown colour where the two fluids meet. The number of C.C. of the uranium solution that have been used is read off; and if, after a second warming of the urine contained in the beaker, and a second trial of the fluid with the solution of the ferrocyanide, no increase in the intensity of the colour be produced, the process may be regarded as completed ; but if a dark brown colour be produced by this second trial, too much uranium solution has been added and the estimation must be begun again with another 50 C.C. of urine.

The calculation for the amount of phosphoric acid passed in twenty-four hours is now easy.

1 C.C. of uranium solution equals 5 milligrammes of phosphoric acid. So that, if 15 C.C. of the uranium solution have been used, 50 C.C. of the urine will contain 75 milligrammes of phosphoric acid, and if the patient have passed 1500 C.C. in the twenty-four hours, the calculation will be :

$$50 : 1500 : : 75 : 2250$$

$$50)\overline{112500}^{75}$$

2250 milligrammes.

2250 milligrammes equal 2·25 grammes, which will be the quantity of phosphoric acid passed in the twenty-four hours.

ESTIMATION OF ALBUMEN.

No easy, rapid, and trustworthy method of estimating albumen has yet been suggested. The ordinary way of coagulating the albumen by heat and acetic acid, throwing the precipitate on a weighed filter, washing, drying, and reweighing, is so long and troublesome that it is never employed in clinical observations.

A fairly good method for clinical observation is the estimation by means of the polariscope. It is necessary to have the urine moderately transparent, and free from blood-corpuscles, sugar, and bile acids, to obtain results which are tolerably accurate. If the turbidity be persistent after filtration, a few drops of acetic acid, or a little carbonate of soda or milk of lime added to the urine before filtration may remove the turbidity. For the method of using the polariscope, see p. 132. See also (p. 26) on the use of Esbach's tubes for clinical determinations.

The quantity of albumen in the urine is usually not more than 1 *per cent.;* it very rarely rises to 4 *per cent.* or more. A patient may pass 2 to 20 grms. of albumen in the twenty-four hours. The latter amount is extreme.

ESTIMATION OF SUGAR.

There are two methods of estimating the amount of sugar present in diabetic urine,

K

one by volumetric analysis, the other by means of the polariscope.

Volumetric Method.—A standard copper solution is required, containing sulphate of copper, neutral tartrate of soda or potash, and solution of caustic soda, 20 C.C. of which correspond to 100 milligrammes of grape sugar. This solution is exceedingly apt to decompose, and must therefore be preserved in well-stoppered, completely filled, glass vessels, and in a cool dark place.

In estimating the sugar, the first step is to ascertain if the copper solution remain undecomposed : it may be used in the analysis, if, after boiling some portion in a test-tube, and setting it aside for an hour, no precipitate of copper oxide have fallen. 20 C.C. of the copper solution are then measured off with a pipette, allowed to flow into a glass flask, and diluted with about 4 times their volume of distilled water. 10 C.C. of the urine are then measured off, and distilled water added until the mixture exactly measure 100 C.C. If, however, the urine contain sugar in but small quantity, it may be diluted with its volume of water only, or indeed with none at all. A burette is filled with the diluted urine, and the flask containing the copper solution is heated over a small flame, wire gauze intervening, until boiling begins; 2 C.C. of the urine are then allowed to flow into the boiling copper solution. After a few seconds, it must be carefully noticed if the copper solution have lost its colour, or be still blue. If it still appear blue when the flask is held between the light and the eye of the observer, another C.C. of the urine must be added to the boiling copper solution; then the colour must be noticed and if it be still blue, the operation should be repeated until the colour of the fluid has become yellow. Where extreme accuracy is required the fluid in the flask must be filtered into three test-tubes, and to the first test-tube a few drops of the copper solution must be added, and the whole boiled to see if an orange-red precipitate of sub-oxide of copper be produced; to the second test-tube a small quantity of hydrochloric acid is then added, and, sulphuretted hydrogen passed through; to the third, acetic acid and ferrocyanide of potassium are added. None of these reagents ought to produce a precipitate.

If, on boiling with the copper solution, a

precipitate occur, too much urine has been added; if, in either of the two last mentioned test-tubes, a precipitate occur, not enough of the urine has been added to decompose all the copper; in either case, the estimation must be repeated.

Since 20 C.C. of the copper solution correspond exactly to 100 milligrammes of sugar, the complete decoloration of the copper solution will be accomplished by exactly 100 milligrammes of sugar. If, therefore, for the 20 C.C. of copper, 15·5 C.C. of the dilute urine were required for complete removal of colour, and if the dilute urine contained only 10 *per cent.* of urine, 1·55 C.C. of urine will contain 100 milligrammes of sugar, and 100 C.C. of urine will contain 6·45 grammes of sugar; as by proportion:

$$1·55 : 100 : : 100 : 6450.$$

If the urine contain albumen as well as sugar, the former must be removed as directed at page 108.

Estimation by means of the Polariscope.—By means of this instrument an estimation of the sugar present can be made, provided that the urine be moderately transparent. If it be passed through animal charcoal, the accur-

acy is greater, of course, but not so great as
to be of much consequence in purely clinical
research. If the urine contain albumen, it
must be removed by the method given above,
page 108. The bile acids when present, can
scarcely affect the result, since they are
found in such very small amount in the urine.

The polariscope consists of a tube, supported upon a foot, and divided into three
parts, one of which, the middle, is movable,
but the other two, which are at the ends of
the instrument, are fixed. One of the fixed
tubes is furnished with a small screw, attached to its lower surface; this may be
called the eye-piece. The other fixed tube
has no screw attached to it; it may be called
the object-glass.

A good argand burner, sodium flame, or a
gas lamp, protected by a neutral tinted glass
cylinder, is necessary. When the polariscope is to be used the lamp is placed an inch
or so in front of the object glass. The hollow glass tube in the middle of the instrument must now be removed, and filled with
distilled water; the small glass disc being
slid over the end of the tube completely filled
with water, in such a manner that no air-

bubble is included in the tube ; the metal
cover to keep the glass disc in its place is
then attached to the tube, and the tube freed
carefully from all moisture. The tube is now
set in its place in the middle of the instrument; and the observer, looking through the
eye-piece, draws out, or pushes in, the move-
able tube close to the eye, until he see at the
end of the eye-piece, nearer to the lamp, a
circular field divided into two equal parts by
a black line, which ought to be sufficiently
well defined. He next turns the screw attached to the under surface of the eye-piece
to the right or left as may be required, until
the colour of the two halves of the field be
exactly the same. The observer then notices
whether the zeroes on the scale above the
eye-piece be exactly opposite to each other.
If they be not, the little button at the end of
the scale should be gently turned, until they
quite coincide.

Before adjusting the instrument, the urine
may be set aside to filter, or to pass through
animal charcoal, if that be at hand. If the
fluid be as free from colour as ordinary diabetic urine, it may be observed in the longer
tube, 20 centimeters in length, since the ac-

curacy of the estimation is increased with the length of the tube. But if the fluid be dark, the shorter tube, 10 centimeters long, must be used.

The tube is now filled with the urine, in the same manner as it was previously filled with distilled water, and again placed in the middle of the instrument. The observer then notices if any alteration in colour of the two halves of the field have taken place. If the uniformity of colour no longer exist, he should turn the screw below the eye-piece until the two halves of the field appear of precisely the same tint. The eyes are best rested occasionally during this part of the operation by looking on some white surface, as the ceiling of the room, or a sheet of paper. When the two semi-circles become exactly the same in colour, the number of degrees which the movable zero is distant from the fixed zero is read off; and if the fluid observed contain sugar, the movable scale will be found to the right; but if albumen only, to the left. The number of degrees that the zero has moved gives when divided by 2, the percentage amount of either sugar or albumen, if the longer tube were used ; but the percentage is at once known, if the shorter tube were employed, as it is the same in amount with the number of degrees by which two zeroes are separated from each other.

INDEX.

www.ingramcontent.com/pod-product-compliance
Lightning Source LLC
Chambersburg PA
CBHW022103210326
41518CB00039B/596